CW00820113

INTERMITTENT FASTING FOR WOMEN OVER 50

The Essential Guide to Lose Weight, Reset
Metabolism and Body Detox

-

Increase your Energy and Rejuvenate your
Body for a Better Life!

LARA WARD

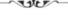

"A diet changes the way you look. A fast changes the way you see."

Lisa Bevere

SUMMARY

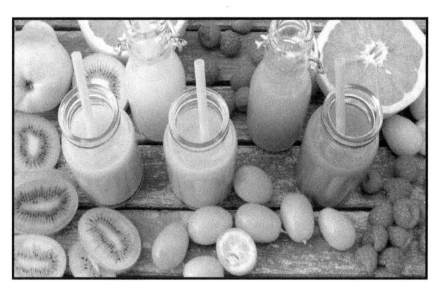

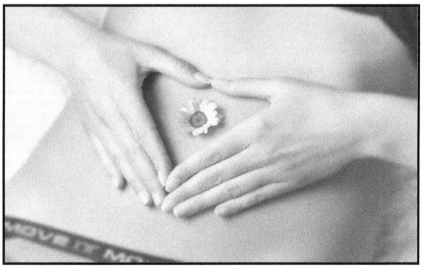

INTRODUCTION

Download for free 15 Low Carb Copycat Recipes for your Intermittent Fasting!

https://bit.ly/2ZsycJY

Intermittent fasting has stood the test of time and is known to have many positive effects in addition to weight loss. We usually forget about the most crucial question when it comes to our diet. We always ask ourselves the question: "What should I eat?" We seem to ask ourselves this question every day, if not several times a day, but what about the question "When should I eat?" It is a much bigger question. This is a question we forgot to ask ourselves.

When we eat, our body produces a hormone called insulin (I'm sure you know that). Insulin determines how what we eat is used. Part of what we eat is used for energy, and part is stored as fat - potential energy. Many of the foods that we consume cause an increase in insulin production, and over an extended period of sustained insulin levels, we begin to develop insulin resistance. At this point, we start to see weight gain and eventually obesity.

Therefore, to avoid insulin resistance, we need to have a

prolonged period of low insulin levels, but how do we achieve this? Well, the answer should be pretty apparent by now. To stop this, we need a period of the complete absence of food. . If all foods increase insulin levels, it follows that no food will automatically lower them. I am talking about "intermittent fasting". It's very different from starvation, so you don't have to ask yourself, "Am I going to starve? Myself?"

Fasting is not dying of hunger. Hunger is an involuntary absence of food. Someone who is starving has no idea when or if the next meal will arrive. There is no control over food consmption. On the other hand, fasting is the voluntary absence of food, whether due to weight loss, religion, or any other reason. The fasting person knows what time to eat again and can eat at any time.

Comparing fasting to starvation is like comparing death by suicide to the end of old age. It's just not the same. Fasting is still an ancient tradition. It is the oldest of all human traditions. Hippocrates considered the father of modern medicine, he said: "To eat when we are sick is to feed our disease".

I'd like to thank you for buying this book. Make sure to leave a short review If you enjoy it, I'd love to hear what you think about it ☺

CHAPTER ONE

UNDERSTANDING INTERMITTENT FASTING

Intermittent fasting (IF) is simply a way to divide your meal plans into mealtimes and fasting times. This innovative fasting model has recently gained popularity among the younger generations. However, the diet has equally essential benefits for older people, especially women. What Are the Benefits of Intermittent Fasting for Women Over 50? Keep reading to find out.

Intermittent fasting for women over 50

This is the age at which women are generally menopausal and postmenopausal; the average age of menopause is 52 years. This is usually accompanied by a shift in body fat from the hips and thighs to the lower abdomen. With lower levels of estrogen, women also lose their protection against heart disease and osteoporosis. Intermittent fasting can help gain weight and fat during menopause and help lower blood cholesterol, blood pressure, insulin resistance, and improve sleep. Although this cohort was not explicitly studied, many of the studies mentioned above included women over 50 in their research.

Benefits of Intermittent Fasting for Women Over 50

Being one of the hottest topics in the weight loss world, intermittent fasting has proven to be an effective remedy for losing weight, maintaining muscle mass, increasing longevity, and improving cognition. Mainly, it is considered to be very useful for older women who want to lose belly fat.

Reduce weight

Belly fat becomes a problem for women as soon as they hit their 40s because of its poor appearance and degrading effects on general health. Weight loss through intermittent fasting allows these postmenopausal women to reduce their risk of various life-threatening illnesses.

Strengthens the musculoskeletal system

Intermittent fasting for women over 50 has been clinically shown to improve overall skeletal system health. It is an effective way to reduce arthritis and back pain symptoms, which older women often experience. Some studies have also shown how changing IF meal plans can affect hormones that control muscle and bone health.

Research has shown that fasting helps reduce the pathways that increase the production of cancer cells. Intermittent fasting for women over 50 can boost self-esteem, improve mood, and reduce negative symptoms like anxiety, depression, and stress.

Controlling diabetes

Eating during specific times is strongly correlated with a lower risk of diabetes. Some studies show that intermittent fasting can be an effective way to control blood sugar, eliminate insulin, and even eliminate or reduce prescription drugs.

Improves longevity

When a woman begins to fast at fixed intervals, her body begins to send a signal that activates the genetic repair mechanism. This mechanism fights aging and other diseases through the production of human growth hormone (HGH). In turn, HGH works to strengthen the muscles, ligaments, and tendons, accelerate metabolism, regenerate tissues and increase longevity. This is perhaps one of the best benefits of intermittent fasting for women over 50.

<u>Types Of Intermittent Fasting</u>

Food limited in time

- A time-limited diet is also called a daily fast. On these fasts, you fast every day and divide the 24-hour day into fasting and eating periods.

- There are popular versions, but you can choose any 24-hour gear to shorten your eating window and lengthen your fasting window from your baseline.

- These are usually written in fasting times - meal times, for example, 2:10 pm, would indicate a 14 hour fast and a meal within 10 hours.

12:12

The main benefit of 12:12 is that it will help you cut down on snacks in the evening after dinner. This is an excellent place to start if your diet is irregular.

16: 8

For this, you can still eat three meals a day. You can use the meal times, such as breakfast at 10:00 am lunch at 2:00 pm, and dinner at 5:30 pm. I should have finished dinner before 6 pm M. So all your food is ready between 10 am M. and 6 pm M., It's been eight hours.

20: 4

With 20 hours of fasting and four hours of meals, you will not eat three meals. You will be more comfortable with two meals or one meal and one snack. It will be easier to achieve this gradually.

OMAD

One meal a day "OMAD" is described as 23: 1, but many people call their eating style OMAD, which means they only eat one meal a day but are not limited to a window. One hour feed. If you want to try OMAD, you should work on it and not start with it.

As I mentioned, these are just a few of the popular fasting / eating windows, you don't have to limit yourself to them, and you don't just need to make one. For example, you can do a 6.10 pm Monday to Thursday and 2.10 pm Friday to Saturday. You may want to build in some flexibility once you've hit your ideal weight and are doing the maintenance. If you have a weight loss goal, you may prefer to keep a shorter feeding window, such as 18: 6.

Weekly fasting regimes

These are based on the number of fasting and feeding days

per week. These are expressed in opposition to time-limited eating, where the days you eat are listed first; For example, eating 4 days and fasting 3 days would be 4: 3.

5: 2

For this, you typically eat five days a week and fast for two days. For the two fasting days, the search used consecutive and non-consecutive days. These are usually not total fat, just water, but low-calorie days, and you would consume about 25% of your calorie needs, usually between 500 and 750 calories per day, and are often referred to as "modified fasts".

ADF

This is the alternative daily fast. As the name suggests, you eat your usual meals one day and fast the next. This is usually a water-only fast, but it can also be changed quickly (500-750 calories). If you think about it in terms of time-limited eating, it's 36:12 where you stop eating after dinner on the first day, say at 7:00 pm, then fast all day two and break your third fast. Day With breakfast at 7:00 am. This would add up to 36 hours of fasting and 12 hours of food or 36:12.

Prolonged fasts

When you fast for more than 48 consecutive hours, it is considered a long fast. It is also called a long fast. Your ghrelin (the hunger hormone) peaks around 6 pm so that you can give up. If you can overcome this, most people report that this third day and beyond is easy. To minimize hunger, you can schedule your fast so that your ghrelin peaks while you sleep. Prolonged fasts should be performed under medical supervision.

Intermittent fasting for women: hormonal balance and crescendo fasting Women are naturally more sensitive to intermittent fasting, possibly due to a chemical called kisspeptin. This sensitivity can cause abnormal periods, disrupt regular cycles, hormonal imbalances in women.

It is essential to keep in mind that no two women are the same. Some do very well with intermittent fasting, and some don't. Should this mean that intermittent fasting is not suggested for those who are sensitive to it? No.

These women should try a milder version of the fast called the Crescendo Rapid. Crescendo Fasting has proven to be the perfect method for middle-aged women over 50 who cannot follow other IF routines and generally have a more challenging time losing weight.

Here is an example for following a crescendo fast:

Perform intermittent fasting twice a week, preferably on non-consecutive days (e.g., Tuesday and Saturday) on an empty stomach for 12 to 14 hours.

Do light physical activities on fasting days, light walks, light yoga, or light aerobics.

Add another quick day after two weeks of IF (e.g., Tuesday, Thursday, and Saturday)

Special Tips For Women Over 50 On Intermitted Fasting

Eat healthy during the meal window.

They say any fool can fast, but it takes intelligence to break it.

What a person eats after breaking a fast is extremely important. The perfect breakfast would contain a large green salad bowl containing raw vegetables dipped in olive oil and steamed broccoli, spinach, or baked yams.

Vegetables are generally preferred because they are easy on the stomach and rich in nutrients. Also, throughout the feeding period, try to maintain a healthy diet with balanced nutrients.

Fiber package

Intermittent fasting for women over 50 can be challenging, especially for those who have not experienced hunger for a few hours each day. Eating foods that are high in fiber and protein while consuming can help combat this problem. Fiber helps a person feel full and can help prevent a drop in blood sugar. Good sources of fiber include whole-wheat bread, pasta, nuts, and beans.

Start with the rapid Crescendo.

Beginner fasts should start with the crescendo method, as it sets more reasonable goals. This is the recommended form of fasting for women because it ensures that hormone levels don't fluctuate too much. Being a much gentler approach to intermittent fasting, this method allows beginners to get the most out of fasting.

Perform regular hormonal checks

Many modified versions of intermittent fasting appear to be safe for women. However, some studies have reported severe side effects like increased hunger, mood swings, reduced focus, bad breath, etc. Some women have also reported a complete interruption of their menstrual cycle by observing the IF. Therefore, it is essential that women who are fasting regularly monitor their hormones. Women are advised to stop fasting immediately if they experience any significant changes in mood or health and contact a doctor.

Additional Weight Loss Tips for Women Over 50

The following tips will help you lose more weight faster.

Get enough sleep

Sleep has a significant impact on the hunger hormones leptin and ghrelin. Ensure you get 6 to 8 hours of sleep a day to regulate your hunger and prevent overeating.

Powertrain

Strength training, weight training, and intermittent fasting will speed up weight loss and increase muscle mass.

Eat less sugar

Sugars or carbohydrates are a significant contributor to weight gain and may decrease the benefits of intermittent fasting. Hence, it is advisable to avoid sugary foods and drinks.

Keep a food journal

Keeping a food journal will help you track your calories and weight loss during the dieting period. This will help you regulate your eating habits and daily schedule as needed and maximize your income.

Take a probiotic

Probiotics are known to improve your digestive health, restore your gut microbiome, and strengthen your immune system. So consider taking probiotic supplements to stay healthy during intermittent fasting.

Intermittent fasting is beneficial for women of all ages. If you're looking to shed those extra pounds and you're a female over 50, try intermittent fasting.

Physiology Of Intermittent Fasting:

How does fasting work

From the necessary understanding, fasting allows our body to shed excess fat. We need to be aware that this fasting process is expected, as many humans have done it repeatedly without any adverse or harmful effects on health. In life, everything is balance.

The good and the bad, yang and yin, apply to fasting and food. Fasting is simply the reversal of eating; therefore, you fast if you do not eat. When we eat food, more energy comes from the food, which cannot be used immediately. Therefore, this energy can be stored for future use. Here, a hormone called insulin plays a vital role in the storage of food energy.

When we eat, the insulin level rises, allowing glucose to be used immediately for energy, but after six hours of eating, the insulin levels begin to drop. At this point, the liver releases glycogen for energy. After 25 to 48 hours of fasting, the liver begins to produce new glucose.

This process is called "Gluconeogenesis" (New Glucose). After 2-3 days of fasting, the body begins a process called "lipolysis" (the breakdown of fat), which burns fat for energy. Here, triglycerides are broken down and used for energy. After five days of fasting, the body begins to produce high levels of human growth hormone (HGH) to maintain muscle mass.

At this point, when all the glucose is used up, we start to burn our fat tissue. This is important because our body cannot burn sugar and fat simultaneously; you can only use one or the other.

The human body is a two-compartment system, which means that there is glucose (sugar) and fat; that is, they are separated. As long as we continue to supply our body with glucose, we will not need to use our fat compartment for energy, even though the glucose is converted into fat deposited in visceral areas of the body, thus increasing obesity.

The only way to get that fat out of the "pool" is to fast, that shift from burning glucose (compartment 1) to burning fat (box 2). Intermittent fasting has been shown to improve insulin insensitivity, which means the longer you fast, the less insulin your body will produce in response to what you eat. Some foods can reduce insulin secretion, and most importantly, they are weak.

Foods are rich in carbohydrates (LCHF). While these foods keep insulin levels low, they do nothing to remedy insulin resistance. This highlights that the remedy for reducing and reversing insulin resistance is to ensure the complete absence of food during specific periods, which can be achieved with fasting. It worked for me, and I guarantee it will work for you.

Five Common Myths And Misconceptions

There are a lot of misconceptions and questions that I hear from people. It is essential to clear them because these myths make people fear fasting because of the dogmas told to them for about fifteen years. This is why it is essential to clarify these myths, and I hope you will learn from them.

Myth # 1: Intermittent Fasting Slows Metabolic Rates:

We have been told that frequent meals boost our metabolism: this is not wrong, but quite the opposite because intermittent fasting within a reasonable amount of time could have done it. Studies have shown that intermittent fasting increases metabolism between 3.6-14%, although many can offset our calories, which is the determining factor if you lose weight.

Myth # 2: Intermittent Fasting Causes Muscle Loss:

This may be true if you do it wrong, but you won't lose muscle if you do it right as long as you eat enough protein for 24 hours or a week. As long as you eat enough and combine it with resistance training and diet, intermittent fasting will never create muscle loss or atrophy because it burns the glycogen stores in your muscles, causing fat to transform. Endogenous in ketone bodies such as acetone.

If your body is burning protein, this is when you lose muscle mass, so you need to understand that as long as you eat enough and have enough fat in your body, you will be fine without worrying about loss Muscular.

Myth 3: Intermittent fasting lowers your testosterone levels:

Like the myth of muscle loss and reduced metabolism, this is entirely wrong. Still, it's a bit more complicated because several studies have shown that testosterone levels decrease after a long fast but increase and even more after weeks of fasting. However, with regular periods of fasting, mostly within 24 hours, fasting increases testosterone levels.

So if you monitor people's testosterone at night when they are adequately fed and then avoid fasting testosterone the next morning, studies have found that testosterone levels increased 20 to 30 times more in the sample. On an empty stomach than in the "fed" state. Testosterone increases with prolonged fasting because fasting is a form of stress on the body. Stress stimulates cortisol levels, which aids in testosterone production and the rise in growth hormone, which maintains muscle mass.

Myth 4: intermittent fasting is bad for women:

This is a common question I hear from women. There is a contradictory opinion of the experts. However, the exact answer is that premenopausal women can experience hormonal changes during intermittent fasting, but this is mostly seen during extremely rapid fasting, hence intermittent fasting.

Mayo is not easy for women because women are more susceptible to stress, and fasting as a body stressor makes some women unable to cope. Many other women fast 20 hours a day, and there is no problem with their hormonal balance.

In short, it depends on the genetic makeup of the woman, as some are more adaptable to the stress associated with intermittent fasting, while others cannot stand it. So it's all up to you. If every day is working well for you: you lose weight, feel energized, and there are no issues with hormonal changes or alterations, then you can. Therefore, it is recommended that you start small and gradually increase your intermittent fasting periods to 21 those that experience some disruption so that your body slowly adapts to the changes.

Myth 5: parry and presume I'm still losing fat:

Intermittent fasting is beneficial when it comes to losing fat. You don't have to start counting calories to see if you're losing weight. All you have to do is avoid processed foods and stick to the usual healthy foods. If you are keen on losing fat fast, combine intermittent fasting with the ketogenic diet, and you will get incredible results.

The Science behind Intermittent Fasting

There is also science involved, which is the production of HGH by your body. Before I get to that, I should explain why this is so. When we eat, our body naturally produces insulin to store carbohydrate glucose for later use. We live in a society where all of our meals are generally regular and bombarded with high levels of sugar and fat in most consumables.

It puts us in an anabolic state, which means we are continually winning. Glucose from food is stored as fat, so you gain weight. Intermittent fasting essentially reverses this process and allows our cells to release stored glucose for energy. The cells enter a catabolic (degradation) state, resulting in weight loss.

HGH is produced in response to your body's need for glucose, so when we always eat, the production of HGH is suppressed because we are getting glucose from it. HGH is responsible for regulating metabolism and has excellent qualities for muscle repair and fat burning. Intermittent fasting has been shown to increase HGH production up to 5 times.

Intermittent Fasting For Longevity

Another aspect of intermittent fasting that I find fascinating and innovative (excuse the term) is its anti-aging effects and the advancements it represents for longevity. This is primarily accomplished through autophagy, which is your body's natural way of cleaning up all damaged cells and replacing them with new, healthy cells. It's like recycling. For longevity, it's fascinating.

A natural and healthy way to replace old cells and get back to producing young cells. Autophagy is programmed into us by our ancestors and works to supplement the body with energy (self-nourishment). It can't go on forever, of course, but you'll be eating every day, so your body doesn't have to go on like this forever. Autophagy increases through intermittent fasting as our cells become stressed.

Autophagy comes into play to help protect and replenish itself. It increases our life expectancy. I love hearing Dr.'s teachings (what's his name?), Who put all these theories into practice on rats. What you have found is amazing. He was able to unequivocally show that CR can increase the lifespan of rats by 30%. No drugs, no drugs, just a simple trick that we can all implement in our lives.

CHAPTER TWO

HOW TO START FOR BEGINNERS

Getting started is easy. Chances are you've tried a lot of intermittent fasting. Many people instinctively eat this way, skipping morning or evening meals. The easiest way to get started is to choose one of the intermittent fasting methods above and try it out.

However, you don't need to follow a structured plan.

An alternative is to fast when it is most convenient for you. Skipping meals now and then when you are not hungry or have no time to cook can work for some people. It doesn't matter what type of fast you choose. The most important thing is to find a method that works best for you and your lifestyle.

Safety and side effects

Modified versions of intermittent fasting appear to be safe for most women. That said, several studies have reported some side effects, including hunger, mood swings, poor focus, reduced energy, headaches, and bad breath on fasting days. There are also stories online from women reporting that their menstrual cycle has stopped after intermittent fasting. If you have a health problem, you should consult your doctor before trying intermittent fasting.

Medical consultation is essential for women who:

You have a history of eating disorders.

- You have diabetes or regularly have low blood sugar.

- They suffer from underweight, malnutrition, or nutritional deficiencies.

- Are you pregnant, breastfeeding, or trying to conceive?

- You have fertility problems or a history of amenorrhea (no periods).

- Intermittent fasting appears to have a good safety profile. However, if you have any issues, such as losing your menstrual cycle, stop immediately.

How to adopt an intermittent fasting diet

Intermittent fasting (IF) is a form of diet and lifestyle change that, instead of drastically reducing calorie intake or eliminating certain food groups, limits the times of day you eat and fast. . Fasting generally includes your hours of sleep and not eating until the end of your fasting period. There are several schemes for implementing an IF regime that you can choose from. FI can be combined with exercise and calorie reduction to reduce inflammation in body tissues and lead to weight loss or muscle gain.

Method a Planning Your Fasting Diet

Consult your doctor before starting an IF diet. Talk to your doctor and explain that you are considering an IF diet. Educate yourself on the pros and cons of the diet, and be sure to let your doctor know about any pre-existing medical conditions.

The IF diet can have a dramatic effect on your daily metabolism. Do not fast without seeing your doctor if you are pregnant or do not feel well.

Warning: Type 1 diabetics on an IF diet would find it difficult to regulate and maintain healthy insulin levels due to deliberately infrequent food consumption.

1. Start with a two-meal window if you are new to fasting. If you are starting an IF diet, plan to eat two healthy meals per day. For example, you could have your first meal at noon and the other at 7:00 pm. Then fast for 17 hours after the second meal, sleeping and skipping breakfast until your fasting period is over.

2. Go for a one-meal period if you can fast for 23 hours. If you have already done so, you might be ready for a stricter plan - if so, set aside a one hour window to eat every day. For example, you can fast for 23 hours and then eat a large, healthy meal between 6 pm and 7 pm every night.

3. Try the 5: 2 diet if it's OK with not eating for a full day. With the 5: 2 diet, eat healthy five days a week and fast for two days. For example, you can eat nothing on Mondays and Thursdays and normally eat (but healthy!) The other five days.

4. Pick a meal schedule that you can stick to. By implementing this diet, you will go without food for repeated periods (for example, fasting 16-23 hours

per 24-hour day) before you start eating for the remaining 1-8 hours of your day. Intermittent fasting is often a way to lose weight, and it's also a great way to regulate and plan your food intake. Establishing and sticking to a daily fasting schedule and setting daily for your last meal at the meal window is essential.

5. Moderately reduce your daily calorie intake. If you usually eat 2,000 or 3,000 calories per day, you can cut calories a bit during meals. Try not to exceed 1,500 or 2,000 calories per day. To achieve this goal, adapt your diet to include healthy carbohydrates, avoid white bread and white noodles, but eat complex carbohydrates and fats.

Eat all of your daily calories for one or two small meals.

You may find that cutting calories is easy to achieve because you simply won't have that much time to consume calories for a week. As part of this process, gradually change your diet to reduce your intake of processed foods, including processed meat, dairy, or soda.

Don't drastically change your diet. When following an IF diet, it is unnecessary to eliminate specific food groups (e.g., carbohydrates or fats). As long as you eat a healthy, balanced diet and don't go over 2,000 calories per day, you can eat the same foods you ate before starting the diet. The IF diet changes you're eating schedule, not the types of foods you eat.

A well-balanced diet includes only small amounts of

processed foods high in sodium and added sugars. Focus on healthy proteins (meats, including poultry and fish), fruits and vegetables, and moderate amounts of daily carbohydrates.

Follow a fasting program

Eat your last meal without fasting. Avoid the temptation to consume junk food, sugar, and processed foods in your last meal before the fast. Eat fresh vegetables and fruits, and make sure you eat plenty of protein to keep your energy levels high. For example, your last meal might include cooked chicken breast, a piece of garlic bread, and a salad that includes romaine lettuce, tomatoes, chopped onions, and dressing.

Some people have a little trouble getting started with this strategy, although it does mean that they will spend more time digesting their food and less time in the "fasting phase" of their food abstinence period. Eat a full meal before starting the fast. If you only fill up on foods high in sugar or carbohydrates before your fast, you will quickly be hungry again. Get plenty of protein and fat when you have a scheduled meal. Cutting back on carbohydrates and fats that are too low can be challenging to maintain as you will feel dissatisfied and always hungry when you fast.

Go on an IF diet. If you are not used to fasting, the IF diet can come as a shock to your appetite and body system. You can join the diet by extending your fasting time between meals or starting with one day off per week. This will benefit your body by allowing your system to detoxify and reduce uncomfortable symptoms (including headaches, low blood pressure, fatigue, or irritability).

Fast during sleeping hours. This will help you not think about stomach growls when you are in the middle of a long fast. Make sure you get at least 8 hours of sleep a night, with at least a few hours of fasting on each side. So, as long as you are awake, you won't feel hungry because you know you can eat a good meal soon.

The first meal / main meal after your fast will be the reward for the fasting period. You will be hungry after the fast, so eat a full meal.

Eat a light snack during your fasting period if necessary. A 100 calorie protein and fat snack (nuts, cheese, etc.) will not affect your fast effectiveness. If you're hungry or starting to feel weak, have a healthy snack! Try to choose snacks with less than 30 calories, such as a few carrots or celery sticks, a quarter of an apple, 3 cherries, raisins or raisins, 2 small cookies, or 1 ounce of chicken or fish until you get the hang of it. 'They are tight.

Keep your body well hydrated. Although you fast most hours of the day on an IF diet, that doesn't mean you should stop drinking. You need to stay hydrated while fasting for your body to function well. Drink water, herbal teas, and other calorie-free drinks. Staying hydrated will also prevent hunger pangs, as fluids will take up space in your stomach.

Lose Weight through an IF Diet

Set yourself a weight loss goal. The IF diet can help you lose weight effectively by reducing your daily calorie intake and allowing your body to burn fat stores. By reducing your time, your body will lose excess body fat by increasing your metabolism. Intermittent fasting can also reduce the amount of inflammation found in body tissue.

Staying motivated to achieve a personal goal through fasting will give you the extra mental strength to keep fasting if you need it. By limiting the time you spend eating, you can reduce excess weight gain. You may be able to extend your life expectancy by burning body fat.

Stay slim and build muscle mass while fasting. An IF diet gives you an excellent opportunity to build muscle. Plan a workout right before your first meal (or, if you eat two meals a day, exercise between meals). Your body will be able to use calories more efficiently at this point, so plan to consume around 60% of your daily calories right after exercise.

To stay healthy and build muscle mass, don't cut calories to less than 10 calories per pound of body weight. For example, a 180-pound man would need at least 1,800 calories per day to lose weight without starving while exercising moderately. Cutting back on too many calories will decrease your ability to stay healthy and build muscle tone.

Adapt your exercise style to achieve the desired body result. The type of exercise you do during an IF diet depends on the product you want. If you are just trying to lose weight, focus on aerobic and cardiovascular exercise. If you're trying to add muscle mass and bulk, you'll need to focus on anaerobic exercises, such as strength training.

If you're trying to lose weight, focus on aerobic or cardiovascular exercise for long sessions. If you want a more muscular body, focus on short periods of anaerobic exercise. Anaerobic media work in short bursts without dramatically increasing your heart rate. It's based on short periods of strength training or weight training, not long aerobic or cardio sessions.

Exercise and Intermittent Fasting: Burn Fat and Build Muscle with IF

Intermittent Fasting (IF) is a diet designed to take the hassle out of counting calories by limiting when you can eat to specific times called "feeding windows." IF has been shown to help you lose and maintain weight, and you can combine it with a healthy exercise regimen to burn even more fat. However, there are several ways to maximize your exercise while following an FI protocol. Fasting can tire you out or exhaust you, but if you feel light-headed, light-headed, or exhausted, stop exercising until you feel better.

Plan your workouts

Do cardio on an empty stomach to burn more fat. Cardiovascular and aerobic exercise uses a lot of energy, and if you fast, your body will draw energy from stored body fat. Burning fat as fuel for your workouts can help you lose weight and reduce the total amount of body fat.

Go for a run or bike ride for a good cardio workout.

Visit your local gym and use the elliptical or rowing machines.

Try group classes in your area to get a little extra motivation by exercising with other people.

Exercise in the morning after getting up to make the time more comfortable. A common and easy way to exercise while fasting is to do it right after waking up, following your body's natural circadian rhythm. Go for a run or bike ride early in the morning to exercise while you are still fasting, which will force your body to extract energy from stored fat, which can reduce overall body fat.

Take a morning class in your gym to start the day right. Suppose you feel too tired or weak to exercise before you eat, don't worry! You can always save your workout for later, during your eating period.

Schedule strength training sessions towards the end of your fast. Resistance training can help prevent muscle loss during an intermittent fasting protocol. Consuming protein an hour after intense strength training can help your muscles recover more effectively. Try to schedule your strength training towards the end of your fast to eat soon after your workout. If your muscles recover better, you may feel less pain the next day.

Track Strength Training With At Least 20 Grams Of Protein - Weight lifting and strength training exercises destroy muscle fibers. Eating at least 20 grams of protein soon after strength training can help maximize muscle protein synthesis, helping you build and maintain muscle mass, which is especially important when cutting calories with a fast Intermittent. After your workout is finished, drink a protein shake or eat lean protein like chicken, tuna, or tofu.

Planning your strength training sessions near you're eating window will allow you to eat protein after your activity is over. Increasing muscle protein synthesis can also help you feel less sore after strength training.

Avoid exercising if you feel faint or dizzy. Although many studies suggest various benefits of intermittent fasting, there is still a lot of science that is not fully known about it. If you experience any unwanted side effects, such as tiredness or dizziness, do not exercise. You could hurt yourself.

Talk to your doctor if you continue to experience side effects from intermittent fasting. Intermittent fasting can be dangerous for people with certain conditions, such as diabetes. Before suddenly making any changes to your diet or lifestyle, talk to your doctor to make sure it's safe for you.

Select Your Ideal Training

Use cardiovascular exercise to lose weight and burn more fat. Aerobic or cardiovascular exercise forces the body to use energy stores as a source of fuel. If you fast, your body will burn fat for energy during your workout. If you are trying to lose weight and body fat, then do some weight training while fasting? Examples of cardiovascular exercise include running, swimming, and cycling.

Strengthen 2-3 times a week to maintain muscle mass. Combining intermittent fasting and exercise is a great way to help you lose weight, but strength training is essential to avoid losing muscle mass. Add strength training or strength training to your weekly exercise regimens.

Studies suggest that you can avoid losing lean muscle mass during intermittent fasting by doing strength training. Because intermittent fasting can reduce the total number of calories you eat per day, you cannot gain strength or increase muscle mass while on a fasting diet.

Avoid HIIT workouts while fasting. High-Intensity Interval Training (HIIT) workouts involve bursts of super-intense exercise, followed by a short rest period. Opt for relatively low-intensity activities while fasting so that your body can recover more efficiently. Stick with the HIIT workouts during your meal period after eating to help you overcome them. If you enjoy HIIT workouts, try a light snack like an energy bar to kick start your meal window and give yourself extra fuel for your workout.

Do a super intense workout only after you eat? Save some long runs, plyometrics, or hefty lifting sessions after eating a meal or two to give yourself enough fuel to finish your workout. Planning your strenuous activities after eating will also help lower your risk of low blood sugar. Track intense workouts with a high-carb snack to help replenish your glycogen stores.

Keep walking if you are fasting for 24 hours. Some fasting protocols involve a full 24 hours of fasting. If you haven't eaten for a full day, stick to very low-intensity exercise, such as walking. Going 24 hours without eating can tire you out, so listen to your body and stop exercising if you feel light-headed or light-headed.

You can also try a beginner's tai chi or yoga class to get your blood pumping without getting exhausted. If you are new to intermittent fasting, you may feel tired and weak, so low-intensity workouts are a good option if you are feeling fatigued.

How To Do An Intermittent "Clean" Fast

Intermittent fasting is a dietary strategy that involves alternating between periods of unrestricted eating, called feeding windows, and fasting periods, limiting the amount of food you eat. A "clean" intermittent fast means that you are only allowed to drink sugar-free, calorie-free beverages, like black coffee and tea, outside of your dining windows. If you are planning on trying intermittent fasting, check with your doctor first to make sure it's safe for you and choose the method that works best for you and your schedule. Even on a "clean" fast, there are a few things you can use to help get you through your fasting periods.

Choose the type of fast

Choose the 16/8 method for a daily feeding window. The 16/8 Protocol, sometimes referred to as the Lean Gains Protocol, means you have an 8-hour window to eat all of your foods every day and fast for the remaining 16 hours. This is one of the most common intermittent fasting methods, and it allows you to eat what you want for a set amount of time each day.

For example, you can set your eating window from noon to 8 pm every day if you don't mind skipping breakfast. You can also choose from 9 to. M. At 5 p. M. Every day otherwise a late snack. The key to the 16/8 protocol is to meet the time limit you set.

Go for the 5: 2 diet to limit your fast to 2 days per week. On the 5: 2 diet, you can usually eat five days a week, but limit yourself to 400-600 calories for two non-consecutive days. This is a good option if you want to limit your fasting periods to just two days a week. For example, you can choose Monday and Thursday as your fasting days, leaving weekends open for everyday eating.

Try alternate day fasting if you can limit yourself to 1 meal on fast days. Alternate fasting means that you alternate between days with no food restriction and days when you have a meal that provides about 25% of your daily calorie needs. If you can organize a dinner party every other day of the week, this may be a good option for you.

So if you are on a 2000 calorie diet, you will eat a 500 calorie meal on fasting days.

An example of an alternate day setting could be to have a meal on Monday, Wednesday, and Friday without any restrictions on other days of the week.

Use plans 4 and 3 for the most extreme option. Also known as a "three-day fast," projects 4 and 3 involve a week consisting of 4 days of unrestricted eating and 3 non-consecutive days in which you fast for a full 24 hours. This is the most challenging option, but it can also have the most health benefits, so it is a good option.

An example of a breakdown may involve fasting on Monday, Wednesday, and Friday, leaving the rest of the week free to eat without restrictions. You cannot consume any calorie-containing food or drink during your fasting days with this model. Talk to your doctor before trying to fast for 24-hour periods to ensure it's safe for you.

Use your eating window to eat until you are satisfied. Whichever method or protocol you choose, it is essential that you use your eating window to fill yourself with enough food to help you get through your next fast. Focus on eating a balanced diet of lean protein, whole grains, and healthy fats to give your body the nutrition it needs. Also, try to avoid processed foods.

Use your meal window to stock up on healthy foods, rather than snacking high in sugar, fat, and salt that don't provide many nutrients, like chips, cookies, and candy.

Control hunger while fasting

Drink enough water to stay hydrated and help reduce food cravings. Water is calorie-free and essential for your body, so you can get as much as you want during your fasting period. Fasting can also make you less thirsty, so you need to drink enough water to avoid dehydration. It is recommended that the average adult drink at least 1.5 liters (0.40 US gallons) of water per day. Remember, on a really "clean" fast; You can't add anything to the water, so avoid lemon wedges and mint leaves.

Drink soda water to avoid feeling hungry. Sparkling water, like sparkling water, is calorie-free and will not break your fast. Plus, the sparkling carbonation can help you feel less hungry. If you experience a persistent feeling of hunger during your fast, try opening some cool soda water. Sparkling water with "natural essences" such as La Croix, Perrier, or San Pellegrino will not break your fast. But if they have any ingredients or added sugar, they will.

Use black coffee to increase energy and reduce hunger. Like black coffee, done calorie-free drinks break your fast and help give you a boost to stay focused and energized. The caffeine in black coffee can also help you feel less hungry while fasting.

However, it must be black coffee. Cream and sugar, even a calorie-free sweetener, will break down you cleanse quickly. Drinking too much caffeine can cause anxiety, tremors, and a rapid heartbeat. Try not to consume more than 500-600 mg of caffeine or about 4-7 cups of coffee.

Try a green, black, or herbal tea as an alternative to coffee. Green tea and black tea contain caffeine, which can lift your spirits if you feel dizzy and reduce your hunger. Studies also suggest that other ingredients in green tea can help you burn fat and reduce hunger. If you don't crave caffeine or are just looking for a flavorful herbal drink, try an herbal tea with no added fruit. Soak a tea bag in 1 cup (240ml) of hot water for about 3 to 5 minutes and enjoy!

Green tea and black tea contain less caffeine than black coffee, so they're less likely to cause nervousness and feel milder on an empty stomach. For example, an 8 A 240 ml (fl oz) cup of black coffee contains about 96 mg of caffeine, while a similar-sized cup of black tea contains about 47 mg. Nuts, herbal teas, such as individual raspberries, blueberries, oranges, or other fruit teas, contain small amounts of sugar that can break the fast.

Drink a glass of apple cider vinegar to reduce cravings. Apple cider vinegar is calorie-free and contains acetic acid, which can reduce your appetite while fasting. Try drinking 1 or 2 teaspoons (4.9-9.9 ml) of apple cider vinegar to suppress appetite if you feel hungry while fasting.

Use apple cider vinegar, not white distilled vinegar.

You can also add apple cider vinegar to a glass of water to dilute the flavor. Exercise to work your body and avoid hunger pangs. Studies suggest that exercising while fasting can increase weight loss, improve body composition, and reduce hunger. If you're hungry, try going for a walk, run, or bike ride. You will burn extra calories, and at the same time, you will avoid being hungry.

Head to your local gym and get on an elliptical trainer or rower.

Sign up for a group fitness class like CrossFit, Zumba, or yoga.

Talk to your doctor if you feel exhausted or sick while fasting. If you have an underlying disease, such as diabetes, or are using medications that require food intake, intermittent fasting may not be safe. Also, if you feel dizzy, exhausted, or dizzy, talk to your doctor. Always talk to your doctor before making any sudden changes to your diet to make sure they are safe for you.

The Basics Of Intermittent Fasting

Eating on an intermittent fast can be as straightforward or as complicated as you are to choose. Some people will continue to eat healthy ahead of time, and others will add another type of diet to it to see results. The ketogenic diet can work very well with this option as it limits your carbohydrates to reduce hunger and burn fat faster. However, you don't need to be on a specific diet to see results when fasting is intermittent.

The first thing to keep in mind is that you cannot eat unhealthy foods when you follow this diet type. It's good to reduce your daytime eating window to eight hours or less (or do one of the other intermittent fasting options). But if you spend that time eating desserts, fast foods, and other unhealthy foods, you will be in trouble.

First, you will not be able to lose weight if you eat this way. Fast foods and other unhealthy options are high in calories per serving, and you will likely eat more than one at a time. Even if you're eating window is smaller, you can still eat too many calories, which will halt any progress in your weight loss. Even though intermittent fasting is not about calorie intake, you should be careful not to eat too many calories. This is an aspect that can affect the effectiveness of intermittent fasting.

You will also notice that when you eat these unhealthy foods, even doing intermittent fasting, it will not improve your health. Your health will depend on a good diet rich in nutrients to stay healthy. Only fasting while eating unhealthy foods is likely to cause as many problems as you had before you started the fast.

When you eat this terrible food, you will find that you are hungry more often and find it challenging to get through your fasting periods. This is because many processed and fast foods contain chemicals and preservatives designed to make you hungry more often. If you want to see results and finish your fast without feeling hungry, now is the time to eat healthier foods.

Now, that doesn't mean you can't eat sweets or junk food

sometimes. Intermittent fasting has no set rules for exactly what you're allowed to eat; you just set the hours you can eat. Eating a small cheat meal is OK, as long as you eat it during your meal times and only do it once in a while. It can be difficult at times, but eating a healthier diet will give you better results.

The trick to doing quick intermittent labor for you is to eat healthily.

The more nutrients you can include in your diet, the better this fast will do for you.

The first thing to consider is to eat a lot of fruit and vegetables. Fresh produce is best because it provides many essential nutrients your body needs to stay healthy. Remember to fill your plate with fruits and vegetables at every meal to get the nutrients you need. Eating a wide variety of foods is also essential to make sure you get what your body needs without adding too many calories.

Then you need to go for good sources of protein. It would be helpful to consider going for options like lean ground beef, turkey, and chicken. Eating bacon and other fatty meats is sometimes OK - don't overdo it. Eating lots of fish will help you get the healthy fatty acids your body needs to function correctly.

Healthy sources of dairy products help you stay lean while giving your body the calcium it needs. You may have a few options like milk and yogurt (be careful with the types that have fruit and other added things as they usually have a lot of sugar), sour cream, cheese, etc. Make sure to control the salts and sugars which are not healthy for the body.

You are allowed to have carbohydrates with this diet. Carbohydrates have gotten a bad rap because many diets recommend that you avoid them.

The important thing here is to eat healthy carbohydrates for you. White bread and pasta are sugars in disguise and should be avoided. To go with whole grain and whole wheat options when it comes to carbs make sure you can get all the nutrition you need.

Eating a well-balanced diet will be the key to feeling good when you are on an intermittent fast. You can mix metals. You choose to get the best results when you do this type of fasting. You are also allowed to have a snack, as long as you are careful this happens often. If you eat junk food, you will be disappointed when you go to the scale and check that you are not losing weight. You can have treats on occasion, but make sure it's not something that diet.

Using the ketogenic diet with intermittent fasting

Many people decide to go on a ketogenic diet while on an intermittent diet fasting to help stay healthy. The ketogenic diet is a moderate protein, high in fat, and a low-carb diet that will help you burn fat fast while reducing your carbohydrate addiction. There is a lot to love with this diet plan, and when it is combined with intermittent fasting, you are sure to get great results just now.

It is possible to use these two regimes together. Intermittent fasting is focused on what times of day you will eat and the ketogenic diet on what eat during these times. For those who want to balance their blood sugar levels and want to lose weight more effectively, by combining these two diet plans together can be significant.

With intermittent fasting, you limit your mealtimes. Instead of spreading out your meals and snacks throughout the day will limit you to just a few hours. Many people will only eat between six and incorporate their macronutrients during this time. Others will take two or three days during the week when they cannot eat and adjust to their nutrients on the other days of the week.

The point is, you limit the time you eat, which forces you to think more about the food you eat. You also benefit from more fat burning and weight loss during intermittent fasting.

During the time you are allowed to eat, you will have to respect the macronutrients we discussed above approved for the ketogenic diet. You will continue with a diet high in fat, moderate in protein, and low in carbohydrates.

Plan even during intermittent fasting. You just need to be more careful on how many times you eat these macronutrients, but you can continue the ketogenic diet is the same. If you want to reap the benefits of intermittent fasting or increase your weight loss, adding this diet to the ketogenic diet can be useful. You can experiment with different log fasting options available to see which one fits your schedule better or work better for you. Of course, if you find that the ketogenic diet is Effective or intermittent fasting is too complicated; you can still stick to it the ketogenic diet, not fast, and see good results.

It is important to remember that it is unnecessary to follow the ketogenic diet if you don't want to do intermittent fasting. Many people choose others to eat healthily rather than going on the ketogenic diet. However, many people will choose to follow the ketogenic diet and intermittent fasting because it is easy to follow and will allow you to lose even more significant.

Eating on an intermittent fast doesn't have to be too difficult. You can choose the foods you want to eat, although it is essential to accompany food that are fresh and whole, and that will fill you up and help you burn fat the process to help you see the weight loss you are looking for.

CHAPTER THREE

TIPS AND SOLUTIONS TO COMMON MISTAKES

10 Tips For Motivation And Success

Try to avoid the sabotage of temptation.

One thing that can put your efforts aside on fast days is the temptation to have other foods in your refrigerator and pantry. If you're relatively sensitive to the visual temptation when it comes to food, you might want to shop for groceries every few days rather than refueling for a week or two. Another thing that may help if you have family members or roommates who are not on the 5: 2 Fast Diet asks them to save all the incredibly tempting prohibited foods.

Organize your refrigerator to make fasting days easier.

Try to allocate the ingredients for the short day on a shelf in the refrigerator. It can help you train your eyes (and your mind) to make only these foods available on fasting days. Over time, you may find that your eyes are not scanning the refrigerator, fixing the foods you cannot eat.

Remember that socialization doesn't have to involve food.

Eating can be an essential part of your social life. Sharing good food or a few drinks with friends and family is part of our culture. However, you can do plenty of other things to have fun on fasting days that don't involve eating.

Focusing on these activities will help you not think about food but avoid having to become a hermit while fasting. Invite friends over to play tennis, attend an art show, spend a day at the beach, or sign up for a dance class with a friend.

If you are a trigger eater, foil the triggers.

Many of us have specific triggers, other than mealtime or hunger, that tell us to eat. Rest at work can automatically send us to the vending machine. Watching television can be likened to snack time. Maybe you tend to pick up leftover dishes from your kids while cleaning the dishes. Go the week before your diet, noting all of the times you snack, then create a plan to deal with those triggers while dieting. Take a break from work a chance to walk for ten minutes. Invite other family members to clean the dishes after dinner. Embroider, cut coupons, stretch a bit, or chew gum while watching TV.

Establish a reward system.

The best way to achieve an important goal is to set several smaller goals and celebrate them as they are achieved. For every couple of days of fasting completed or every pound lost, treat yourself to a little treat. It could be a manicure, a new book, a movie night with your spouse, or just an hour for you in the park.

Include your friends and family on your team.

Let friends and family know that you are on an empty stomach diet and give them an idea of the guidelines. Even if they don't support the diet, they can still help you out by telling you how good-looking it is and not showing up to your house with a dozen donuts.

Partner.

One of the most motivating things you can have when you start a diet is to have someone do it with you. Find a coworker, friend, or family member who is interested in trying the 5: 2 Quick Diet so that you can support and encourage each other.

Take it one day at a time.

Sometimes just the thought of dieting for an entire month can overwhelm you. Try to focus on one day at a time. Take this attitude: "I don't have to stick to my diet tomorrow, I just have to stick to today." Of course, you will repeat it every day!

Learn to distinguish between hunger and other feelings.

Most of us eat a lot without thinking. We eat because we are angry, eat because we are bored, or eat because we are tired. Start taking note of your feelings every time you think about eating something. You may find that you just need to move around most of the time, talk to a friend on the phone, or go to bed.

If you are hungry, drink water.

It is often difficult to tell the difference between thirst and hunger. Whenever you feel the need for a snack, drink a glass of water. Hunger pains can go away most of the time.

Common Mistakes and How to Avoid Them

You don't relax on it.

You are skipping breakfast. Skip lunch. And at 3 p.m. you are ready to eat your arm. "If you normally eat every 3-4 hours and then suddenly shorten your eating period to 8 hours, you're probably hungry all the time and discouraged," said Libby Mills, RD, dietitian at Villanova University's College. . of nursing.

"The decision to limit your meals may be motivated by weight loss. However, this is an opportunity to familiarize yourself with how your body really feels. We often eat every 3-4 hours and not always because we are hungry." You don't have to fast all week either. In fact, people on the 5: 2 diet eat regular amounts of healthy foods for 5 days and flip the switch on the other 2 days, reducing their calorie intake. A study of 107 overweight or obese women found that women who cut calories twice a week lost as much as women who consistently cut calories.

You consume too many calories.

According to Mills, you're not alone. "It can be easy to overeat when you break a fast, either because you're hungry or justifying yourself to make up for lost calories." She recommends using a scale of 0 to 10, where 0 means hunger and 10 is full. You need to be hungry before you eat and you should stop eating when you're full, not just to clean your plate. He also recommends slowing down while eating so your brain has time to see when it gets full. "It can take 15 to 20 minutes after you start eating," says Mills.

You sabotage with soda.

Mills says the carbonation in soda can mask your hunger pangs, which can lead to you being overly hungry at your next meal and overeating. "Artificially sweetened drinks can also increase the satisfaction of sweet flavors, so if you eat a piece of fruit, it may not satisfy you.

He adds that these drinks can also contain caffeine, which can affect people differently. "A little caffeine can make you nervous and lead to sweet cravings. While other caffeine can mask your hunger pangs and delay it until the hunger is over."

It does not track your water consumption.

In general, you should drink 2 liters (i.e., 1/2 gallon) of water per day. "Water is part of our body's metabolic responses and is necessary for it to function properly. Hydration prevents us from confusing hunger with thirst," Mills notes.

When snacking, opt for non-starchy fruits and vegetables that contain water (yes, hydrating foods count towards your daily water goal!). Make sliced cucumbers, celery, watermelon, and oranges in the fridge or lunch box.

You are not eating the right foods when you break your fast.

Mills says eating enough lean protein (such as meat, poultry, fish, and vegetable proteins such as legumes), nuts, and seeds with each of your meals will help you feel full for longer. "Protein helps us feel full. Plus, when you lose a few pounds, protein helps keep your lean body mass metabolically active."

Another benefit, according to Mills, is that the fiber in fruits, vegetables, whole grains, and legumes slows down the digestion and absorption of the carbohydrates you eat, so you can stay full and energized longer between meals. "Even when you choose foods that contain protein and fiber, you get the vitamins, minerals and nutrients you need while redistributing your calorie intake."

Your approach is too extreme.

Sure, you want to grab this diet trend by the lapels and run with it, but there's no need to starve yourself. Eating less than 800 calories per day will lead to more weight loss (with a significant increase in hunger) but more bone loss. That is not healthy, nor sustainable, in the long term. Not to mention, if you manage to keep your windows from eating too long, you won't be able to continue like this. Make smaller, more manageable changes, and always listen to your body.

You have caffeine withdrawal.

Who said ditch your morning Joe, afternoon espresso, or hot tea? None! In fact, coffee is not bad for you. Mills says that "a caffeinated drink, especially if it's hot, is a comforting bridge between meals." Remember, do not add sugar or milk if you drink your cup when you are fasting.

You are in your own head.

Whether you stick with intermittent fasting for a week or a month, it should feel like a natural part of your routine. "Shifting your focus to be more intuitive about when you eat based on your feelings of hunger and satiety makes sense for a lifetime."

"Choosing foods that nourish your body with the nutrients it needs to stay energized shifts the mindset from counting calories to a focus on quality of life." It is less a model of diet and more of a new way of thinking and consuming food.

Participate in intense and hard training.

You can exercise, but not like the Hulk. It's hard to do your best in a workout if your tank is empty. Moderate exercise is important for health benefits, but if you want to exert yourself a little more, make sure you don't have hours to go before your next meal. Basically, don't go to the gym at 5 a.m. and don't break your fast until 2 p.m. Your body needs fuel to get through a tough workout and replenish its reserves after one.

You give up because you ate at the wrong time.

Don't throw in the towel, and don't beat yourself up. You don't undo all your work with one meal, but you can do it with a bad attitude. Take the time to reevaluate and make sure the schedule you have set continues to work with your lifestyle. Maybe you don't anymore and want to change your eating window or relax it a bit. It's okay. Also, you recovered by concentrating on your food choices and eating as many high-quality, nutritious foods as possible. If you have the right balance of protein, fiber, non-starchy vegetables, and H2O, you won't be hungry throughout the day.

Talk to everyone about intermittent fasting.

It is normal to want to talk about something new that you are excited to learn. However, understand that many people may not approve of intermittent fasting. They may try to discourage you and convince you not to try. Some misinformed friends may feel like it will ruin your hormones or put you in the way of eating a mess.

Never change things

To find the best intermittent fasting method, you will probably need to experiment a bit. Once you experience the results you are looking for, it can still be helpful to make changes from time to time. For example, if, like me, you feel that the warrior's diet is optimal, you can still benefit from a 24-hour fast every now and then. Or maybe a modified fast several times a year. It is often a good idea to change your method from time to time.

Eating too many carbohydrates.

A moderate amount of carbohydrates (between 50 and 200 grams per day) is optimal for most women. If you regularly eat more than 200 grams per day, it can be more difficult to fast. Sometimes on the weekend, I take a break from the intermittent fast. That one day, I can eat paleo pancakes for breakfast, put honey in my coffee, eat desserts, etc. I probably have more than 200 grams of carbohydrates, and it gets harder and harder to fast the next day. Keeping your carbohydrate intake low will make fasting easier.

If fasting is too hard, your hunger is affecting your behavior, and you feel like you can't continue, try testing your ketones to see if you're making ketones. Ketosis makes fasting possible. If you can't get into ketosis, you should eat fewer carbohydrates.

Don't learn to tell the hunger signals.

I would like to emphasize that fasting is not just about turning off hunger signals. It's about learning to distinguish them. With practice, you will notice the difference between regular hunger, which is just a slightly uncomfortable feeling in your stomach, and hunger that you should honor, which makes you feel weak or hungry.

Some days I can go without food until 5 pm because I feel really good and the hunger doesn't bother me. Other days I decide to have an avocado or a whole salad for lunch because I don't feel so good and can't go on like this. Now I can do this with confidence because through practice, and I have been able to feel the difference.

Compare yourself with others.

It may take longer than expected to reach your goals. If you see someone else getting more obvious results than you, it doesn't mean that intermittent fasting won't work for you. It just means that your body reacts differently. Learn to focus on what you are accomplishing and don't let the success of others put you off.

Eating junk food instead of nutrient-rich foods.

Whether you practice intermittent fasting or not, it is always important to choose your foods wisely. Consuming whole foods rich in nutrients promotes optimal health. I recommend that you make vegetables the majority of your diet. Add proteins, healthy fats, grains, and legumes if necessary.

- Are you enjoying *Intermittent Fasting for Women over 50*? If so, I'd really appreciate if you could leave a short review.. It means a lot to me! Thank you so much. -

CHAPTER FOUR

RECIPES FOR FASTING DAYS

Note on Fast Day Recipes: All Fast Day recipes were created to make two servings. If you don't have a friend or family member on the Fast 5: 2 diet with you, simply cut the recipe in half or save the second serving for another meal.

GREEK BREAKFAST WRAPS
(250 calories per serving)

This recipe is just as satisfying as this fast-food breakfast sandwich, but this wrapper has a lot less fat and fewer calories. It's a great breakfast to make ahead and warm up in the morning or at work.

Ingredients:

- 1 teaspoon of olive oil

- ½ cup of fresh spinach leaves

- 1 tablespoon of fresh basil

- 4 beaten egg whites

- ½ teaspoon of salt

- ¼ teaspoon freshly ground black pepper

- ¼ cup crumbled low-fat feta cheese

- 2 whole wheat tortillas (8 inches)

Instructions:

1. In a small pan, heat olive oil over medium heat. Add the spinach and basil to the pan and sauté for about 2 minutes or until the spinach is softened.

2. Add the whites to the pan, season with salt and pepper, and sauté, often stirring, for about 2 minutes more, or until the whites are set.

3. Remove from heat and sprinkle with feta cheese.

4. Microwave tortillas for 20 to 30 seconds, or until tender and warm. Divide the eggs between the tortillas and wrap them like a burrito.

5. Makes 2 servings.

TOMATO PARMESAN EGG TOAST
(150 calories per serving)

This breakfast is quick to make and delicious to eat. You can substitute grape tomatoes if you have them on hand. They provide a good dose of vitamin C in your meal.

Ingredients:

- 1 teaspoon of olive oil

- ½ teaspoon minced garlic (about 1 clove)

- 6 cherry tomatoes, cut into wedges

- ½ teaspoon of salt

- ¼ teaspoon freshly ground black pepper

- 2 large eggs

- 2 slices of low-calorie whole wheat toast

- 1 tablespoon of grated Parmesan

Instructions:

1. In a small pan, heat olive oil over medium heat. Add garlic and tomatoes to the pan and sauté for 2 minutes, stirring frequently. Season with salt and pepper, then transfer to a plate to keep warm.

2. In the same pan, brown the eggs for 2 minutes. Flip and cook until cooked through (30 seconds for easy, 1 minute for too medium, 2 minutes for too good).

3. Place 1 egg on each toast, top with half the tomatoes, and sprinkle with half the Parmesan.

4. Makes 2 servings.

CURRY CHICKEN BREAST WRAPS
(250 calories per serving)

These quick, filling wraps offer lots of flavor for very few calories. Prepare the topping ahead of time, so you have it on hand for working lunches and busy days.

Ingredients:

- 6 ounces of cooked chicken breast, cubed

- 2 tablespoons of low-fat plain yogurt

- 1 teaspoon of Dijon mustard

- ½ teaspoon of mild curry powder

- 1 small Gala or Granny Smith apple, cored and chopped

- 1 cup mixed spring lettuce or tender lettuce

- 2 whole wheat tortillas (8 inches)

Instructions:

1. In a small bowl, combine the chicken, yogurt, Dijon mustard, and curry powder; mix well to combine. Add apple and stir until blended.

2. Divide the lettuce among the tortillas and top each with half the chicken mixture. Roll up burrito-style and serve.

3. Makes 2 servings.

BAKED SALMON FILLETS WITH TOMATOES AND MUSHROOMS (200 calories per serving)

Salmon is an excellent source of healthy fats, especially omega-3 fatty acids. When cooked with a mixture of spicy tomatoes and wild mushrooms, it is as delicious as it is healthy.

Ingredients:

- 2 salmon fillets with skin (4 ounces) • ½ teaspoon of chopped fresh dill

- 2 teaspoons of olive oil, divided • ½ cup fresh tomato, diced

- ½ teaspoon of salt • ½ cup of sliced fresh mushrooms

- ¼ teaspoon of freshly ground black

Instructions:

1. Pepper

2. Preheat the oven to 375 degrees F and line a baking sheet with foil.

3. Using your fingers or a pastry brush, coat both sides of the fillets with ½ teaspoon of olive oil each. Place the salmon skin-side down in the pan. Sprinkle evenly with salt and pepper.

4. In a small bowl, combine the remaining 1 teaspoon of olive oil, dill, tomato, and mushrooms; mix well to combine. Pour the mixture over the fillets.

5. Fold the foil's sides and ends to seal the fish, place the pan on the middle rack of the oven and bake for about 20 minutes, or until the salmon flakes easily.

6. Makes 2 servings.

SWEET POTATO PROTEIN ENERGY
(200 Calories per Serving)

This recipe is quick and straightforward, but it has almost ten grams of protein per serving, making it a perfect quick meal to keep you full and keep you going and concentrated.

Ingredients:

- 2 medium sweet potatoes

- 6 ounces of plain Greek yogurt

- ½ teaspoon of salt

- 1/3 cup dried cranberries

- ¼ teaspoon freshly ground black pepper

Instructions:

Instructions:

1. Preheat the oven to 400 degrees F and pierce the sweet potatoes a few times with a fork. Place them on a baking sheet and bake for 40 to 45 minutes, or until they can be easily pierced with a fork.

2. Cut the potatoes in half and pour the pulp into a medium bowl, keeping the skin intact. Add salt, pepper, yogurt, and blueberries to the bowl and mix well with a fork.

3. Pour the mixture into the skin of the potatoes and serve hot.

4. Makes 2 servings.

AVOCADO FENNEL SALAD WITH BALSAMIC VINAIGRETTE (150 calories per serving)

This salad is a lovely blend of tangy citrus and silky fennel flavored with anise and avocado. Tossed with a quick and easy balsamic vinaigrette, it's a perfect light lunch or dinner for hot days.

Ingredients:

- 1 tablespoon of light olive oil

- ½ cup fennel, sliced

- 1 tablespoon of balsamic vinegar

- ½ avocado, diced

- teaspoon of salt

- cup of tangerines, drained

- 1 cup chopped romaine lettuce

- ¼ teaspoon freshly ground black pepper

1. In a medium bowl, combine olive oil, balsamic vinegar, salt, and pepper and whisk until well combined and slightly thick. Here is your balsamic vinaigrette.

2. Add the fennel, avocado, oranges, and lettuce; Stir until the vegetables are coated with the dressing. Divide between two salad plates and serve cold.

3. Makes 2 servings.

PENNE PASTA WITH VEGETABLES
(200 calories per serving)

Even on fasting days, you can enjoy a light pasta meal. This one is packed with vitamin C and iron from spinach and tomatoes and offers a lot of flavor and satisfaction.

Ingredients:

- 1 teaspoon of salt, divided

- ¾ cup uncooked penne pasta

- 1 tablespoon of olive oil

- 1 tablespoon minced garlic

- 1 teaspoon of fresh oregano, minced

- 1 cup sliced fresh mushrooms

- 10 cherry tomatoes, cut in half

- 1 cup of fresh spinach leaves

- ½ teaspoon of freshly ground black pepper

- 1 tablespoon of grated Parmesan

Instructions:

1. In a large saucepan, bring 1 liter of water to a boil. Add ½ teaspoon of salt and a pen, cook according to package directions, or until al dente (about 9 minutes). Drain the pen, but do not rinse it, reserving about ¼ cup of pasta water.

2. Meanwhile, in a large skillet, heat olive oil over medium-high heat. Add garlic, oregano, and mushrooms and sauté for 4 to 5 minutes or until mushrooms are golden brown.

3. Add the tomatoes and spinach, season with the remaining ½ teaspoon of salt and black pepper, and sauté for 3 to 4 minutes, or until the spinach is tender.

4. Add the drained pasta to the pan, along with 2-3 tablespoons of pasta water. Cook, constantly stirring,

for 2 to 3 minutes, or until pasta is shiny and water is cooked through.

5. Divide the pasta between two shallow bowls and sprinkle with Parmesan cheese. Serve hot or at room temperature.

6. Makes 2 servings.

HEARTY SHRIMP AND KALE SOUP
(250 calories per serving)

This flavorful soup is packed with antioxidants from carrots and kale, as well as a fair amount of shrimp and bean protein. It's delicious, simple, and satisfying.

Ingredients:

- 1 teaspoon of olive oil

- 2 cloves garlic

- ¼ cup onion, minced

- 2 cups chopped fresh kale

- 1 cup finely sliced fresh carrots

- ½ teaspoon of salt

- 1½ cup of vegetable broth

- 8 medium raw shrimps (36 to 40), peeled and cut in half

- 1 cup canned large northern beans, drained

- ¼ cup chopped fresh parsle

- ¼ teaspoon freshly ground black pepper

Instructions:

1. In a medium saucepan, heat olive oil over medium heat. Add garlic, onion, kale, carrots, and sauté for 5 minutes, stirring frequently.

2. Season the vegetables with salt and pepper, then add the vegetable broth.

3. Simmer, uncovered, 30 minutes or until carrots are tender.

4. Increase the heat and bring the soup to a boil. Add the shrimp and cook for 2 minutes, or until the shrimp are pink and slightly firm. Reduce the heat to a minimum.

5. Use a fork to mash about a quarter of the beans. Add all the beans to the soup and add the parsley. Cook over low heat for 2 minutes or until heated through.

6. Serve in soup bowls and serve hot.

7. Makes 2 servings.

PORK LOIN CHOPS WITH MANGO SAUCE
(250 calories per serving)

This recipe is bursting with flavor and satisfying enough to make you forget you're fasting. The sauce is even better a day ahead, so marinate it in the fridge overnight with the pork chops.

Ingredients:

- 2 ¾ inch thick pork chops
- ½ cup diced green pepper
- ½ cup of lemon juice
- ½ cup diced red pepper
- the juice of a large orange
- 1 small jalapeño pepper, seeded
- 1 large freshly ripe mango, peeled and diced
- 1 tablespoon of chopped fresh coriander
- ½ cup red onion, chopped
- 1 tablespoon of chopped fresh parsley
- ½ teaspoon of salt
- ¼ teaspoon of freshly ground black
- Pepper

Instructions:

1. Place the pork chops in a freezer bag and add the lime and orange juice. Seal, shake to mix well and place in the refrigerator overnight.

2. In a small bowl, combine the mango, red onion, peppers, jalapeño peppers, cilantro, and parsley. Stir to mix well. Cover and refrigerate overnight.

3. Preheat the grill and line a baking sheet with foil.

4. Season each pork chop on both sides with S&P. Place the pan and grill for 4-5 minutes on one side, then flip and grill for an additional 4-5 minutes. Place each pork chop on a plate, pour the sauce over it and serve.

5. Makes 2 servings.

SESAME CHICKEN WITH LEMON AND ASPARAGUS (200 calories per serving)

Chicken and asparagus combine wonderfully. This recipe combines them with a touch of lemon and the added crunch of sesame seeds.

Ingredients:

- 8 ounces of skinless chicken breast (or chicken breast cut into quarters) • ½ cup plus 1 tbsp lemon juice, divided

- 1 teaspoon of chopped fresh rosemary

- 6 medium-sized fresh asparagus, cut into 2-inch pieces

- ½ teaspoon of olive oil

- 1 teaspoon of salt, divided

- 2 tablespoons of sesame seeds

- ¼ teaspoon freshly ground black pepper

Instructions:

1. Mash the chicken fillets with a mallet or the palm of

your hand until they are a uniform ½ inch thick. Place in a freezer bag with ½ cup lemon juice and marinate for 2 hours or overnight.

2. Preheat the grill and line a baking sheet with foil.

3. Season the chicken on both sides with ½ teaspoon of salt and pepper and place it in the pan. Sprinkle with rosemary.

4. In a small bowl, toss the asparagus with the olive oil, the remaining tablespoon of lemon juice, and the remaining ½ teaspoon salt. Place the asparagus around the chicken in the pan.

5. Grill the chicken for 4 to 5 minutes, then turn it over, stir in the asparagus, and grill 4 to 5 minutes more.

6. Divide the chicken and asparagus between two plates and sprinkle with sesame seeds.

7. Makes 2 servings.

SPINACH AND SWISS CHEESE OMELET
(150 calories per serving)

No need to reserve omelets for breakfast or brunch. An omelet can be a great dinner solution on busy evenings and makes a satisfying starter for lunch on weekends.

Ingredients:

- 1 teaspoon of olive oil

- 6 large egg whites, beaten

- 1 cup of fresh spinach leaves

- ½ teaspoon of salt

- ¼ teaspoon freshly ground black pepper

- 2 slices (1 oz) of low-fat Swiss cheese

Instructions:

1. In a small skillet, heat olive oil over medium-high heat. Add the spinach, salt, and pepper and sauté for 3 minutes, stirring frequently.

2. Use a spatula to distribute the spinach reasonably evenly over the pan's bottom and pour the egg whites on top, tilting the pan to cover the spinach thoroughly.

3. Cook for 3 to 4 minutes, occasionally pulling the edges of the eggs towards the center while tilting the pan to allow the raw egg to spread around the edges of the pan.

4. When the center of the eggs is mostly (but not wholly) dry, use a spatula to turn the eggs. Place the Swiss cheese slices in one half of the tortilla, then scan the other half on top to form a croissant. Cook 1 minute or until cheese is melted and heated through.

5. To serve, cut the tortilla in half and serve hot.

6. Makes 2 servings.

GRILLED CHICKEN SALAD WITH POPPY SEED DRESSING

(200 calories per serving) Salads are easy to prepare, and

when made with lots of fresh vegetables and high in fiber, they provide a lot of nourishment for very few calories. This salad not only tastes great, but it also fills you up nicely.

Ingredients:

- 2 tablespoons of light olive oil

- 1 tablespoon of apple cider vinegar

- 1 teaspoon of Dijon mustard

- 1 tablespoon of poppy seeds

- ½ cup minced cooked chicken breast

- 1 cup chopped romaine lettuce

- 1 medium cucumber, unpeeled, sliced

- 1 medium red pepper, chopped

- 1 small red onion, minced

Instructions:

1. In a medium bowl, whisk together olive oil, apple cider vinegar, Dijon mustard, and poppy seeds for about 1 minute, or until blended and smooth.

2. Add the chicken, lettuce, cucumber, bell pepper, and onion and mix well until evenly coated.

3. Divide between two salad plates and serve immediately.

4. Makes 2 servings.

QUICK MISO SOUP WITH BOK CHOY AND SHRIMP
(150 calories per serving)

If you like Asian flavors, you'll love this quick and easy soup. It comes together in minutes, making it an excellent recipe for your busiest nights. It heats up nicely, which also makes it the right choice for a working lunch.

Ingredients:

- 2 cups of water

- 8 large raw shrimps (34 to 40 units), peeled and cut in half

- 1 cup minced bok choy

- ¼ cup white miso paste

- 1 cup cubed firm tofu

- 2 green onions, chopped

Instructions:

1. In a medium saucepan, bring water to a boil over high heat. Add the shrimp and boil for 1 minute.

2. Reduce the heat to low and add the bok choy. Simmer for 2 minutes, then add the miso and tofu. Cook over low heat for 1 more minute.

3. To serve, divide between two bowls and sprinkle with chives.

4. Makes 2 servings.

ROASTED HALIBUT WITH GARLIC SPINACH
(200 calories per serving)

Halibut is a deliciously moist fish loaded with heart-healthy omega-3 fatty acids. If you are replacing frozen Halibut, be sure to thaw and dry it thoroughly before cooking.

Ingredients:

- 2 halibut fillets (4 ounces) 1 inch thick

- ½ lemon (about 1 teaspoon of juice)

- 1 teaspoon of salt, divided

- ¼ teaspoon freshly ground black pepper

- ½ teaspoon of cayenne pepper

- 1 teaspoon of olive oil

- 2 cloves garlic

- ½ cup red onion, chopped

- 2 cups of fresh spinach leaves

Instructions:

1. Preheat the grill and place an oven rack 4 to 5 inches below the heat source.

2. Cover a baking sheet with foil.

3. Squeeze half a lemon over the fish fillets, then season each side with ½ teaspoon of salt, pepper, and cayenne pepper. Place the fish in the pan and grill for

7 to 8 minutes. Turn the fish over and grill for an additional 6-7 minutes, or until flaky.

4. Meanwhile, heat the olive oil in a small skillet over medium heat. Add the garlic and onion and sauté for 2 minutes. Add the spinach and the remaining ½ teaspoon of salt and sauté for two more minutes. Remove from heat and cover to keep warm.

5. To serve, divide the spinach between two plates and garnish each serving with a fish fillet. Serve hot.

6. Makes 2 servings.

CURRIED BLACK BEAN & SWEET POTATO QUINOA (250 calories per serving)

Beans, quinoa, and sweet potatoes combine to provide a healthy, filling serving of meatless protein that's so satisfying. You can prepare the quinoa in the microwave if you prefer; follow the package's directions to get a mug.

Ingredients:

- ½ cup of quinoa

- 1 cup of water

- ½ cup sweet potato, peeled and diced (about 1 small)

- ½ teaspoon of olive oil

- ½ teaspoon of dried rosemary

- 1 cup canned black beans, drained

- 1 teaspoon of mild curry powder

- 2 tablespoons of chopped fresh parsley

Instructions:

1. Rinse the quinoa under cold running water in a fine colander. Drain well on absorbent paper, then pat dry.

2. In a small saucepan, toast the quinoa for 2 minutes over medium heat, stirring frequently. Add the water, increase the heat to high and bring the water to a boil. Cover, reduce heat to low, and cook for 15 minutes or until

3. 4 thin slices of fresh tomato

4. Quinoa is thick, and the germ forms small spirals in each grain. Remove from heat and cover to keep warm.

5. In a small bowl, toss the sweet potato with olive oil and rosemary. Transfer to a medium skillet over medium-high heat. Sauté, stirring frequently, 6 to 7 minutes, or until well caramelized. Add the black beans and curry powder, reduce the heat to medium, and cook, frequently stirring, until the beans are heated through.

6. To serve, place ½ cup of cooked quinoa on each plate and top with half the bean mixture. Garnish with parsley.

7. Makes 2 servings.

GRILLED PEPPER SANDWICHES
(150 calories per serving)

Grilling, rather than grilling, your cheese sandwich adds tons of satisfying crunch while omitting the extra fat. These grilled cheese sandwiches are packed with lots of heat in every bite.

Ingredients:

- 2 low-calorie red pepper slices

- ½ cup fresh arugula leaves cheese

- 4 slices of low-calorie whole wheat bread

Instructions:

1. Preheat the oven to 350 degrees F.

2. Place 1 slice of cheese on each of the two slices of bread; top each with two tomato wedges and half the arugula. Top with remaining slices of bread and place sandwiches on a baking sheet in the center of the oven.

3. Broil for 4 minutes, then turn and broil for 2-3 more minutes, or until bread is golden brown and cheese is melted. Cut each sandwich in half for serving.

4. Makes 2 servings.

FAST BOK CHOY SHRIMP MISO SOUP
(150 calories per serving)

If you like Asian flavors, you will love this simple and quick soup. It comes together in just a few minutes, making it a great recipe for your busiest nights. It heats up well, which makes it a good choice for a weekday lunch as well.

Ingredients:

- 2 cups of water

- XA cup of white miso paste

- 8 large raw shrimps (34-40 pieces),

- 1 cup of firm diced tofu

- peeled and cut in half

- 2 green onions, chopped

- 1 cup of chopped bok choy

Instructions:

1. In a medium saucepan, bring the water to a boil over high heat. Add the shrimp and cook for 1 minute.

2. Lower the heat and add the bok choy. Simmer for 2 minutes, and then add the miso and tofu—Cook for another minute on low heat.

3. To serve, divide between two bowls and sprinkle with chives. Makes two servings.

ROASTED HALIBUT WITH GARLIC SPINACH
(200 calories per serving)

Halibut is a deliciously moist fish that is packed with heart-healthy omega-3 fatty acids. If you are replacing frozen halibut, be sure to thaw it completely and dry it thoroughly before cooking.

Preheat the grill and place an oven rack 4-5 inches below the heat source. Cover a baking tray with aluminum foil.

Ingredients:

- 2 halibut fillets (4 ounces) 2.5 cm thick

- Lemon V2 (about 1 teaspoon of juice)

- 1 teaspoon of salt, divided

- 4 teaspoons of freshly ground black pepper

- V2 teaspoon of cayenne pepper

- 1 teaspoon of olive oil

- 2 cloves of garlic

- V cup red onion, chopped

- 2 cups of fresh spinach leaves

Instructions:

1. Squeeze half a lemon over the fish fillets and season with a teaspoon of salt, pepper, and cayenne pepper on each side. Place the fish in the pan and grill for 7 to 8 minutes. Flip the fish over and grill for another 6 to 7 minutes, or until flaky.

2. Meanwhile, heat the olive oil in a small frying pan over medium heat. Add the garlic and onion and fry for 2 minutes. Add the spinach and the remaining teaspoon of salt and cook for 2 more minutes. Remove from

heat and cover to keep warm.

3. Before serving, divide the spinach between two plates and cover each portion with a fish fillet. Serve hot.

4. Makes 2 servings.

QUINOA WITH BLACK BEANS AND SWEET POTATOES (250 calories per serving)

Beans, quinoa, and sweet potatoes combine to make a healthy, hearty serving of meatless protein that is so satisfying. You can prepare the quinoa in the microwave if desired; just follow the directions on the package to get a mug.

Rinse the quinoa under cold running water in a fine-mesh strainer. Drain well on kitchen paper and pat dry.

Ingredients:

- V2 cup of quinoa

- 1 cup of water

- V cup sweet potato, peeled and diced (about 1 small)

- V teaspoon of olive oil

- V teaspoon of dried rosemary

- 1 cup of canned black beans, drained

- 1 teaspoon of mild curry powder

- 2 tablespoons of fresh parsley, finely chopped

Instructions:

1. Roast the quinoa in a small saucepan over medium heat for 2 minutes, stirring frequently. Add the water, turn up the heat and bring the water to a boil. Cover, reduce heat and cook for 15 minutes, or until the quinoa is thick and the germ forms small spirals in each grain. Remove from heat and cover to keep warm.

2. In a small bowl, mix the sweet potato with olive oil and rosemary.

3. Transfer to a medium skillet over medium heat. Sauté, frequently stirring, for 6 to 7 minutes, or until well caramelized. Add black beans and curry powder, reduce heat to medium, and cook, frequently stirring, until beans are heated through.

4. To serve, place your V2 cup of cooked quinoa on each plate and cover with half of the bean mixture. Garnish with parsley.

5. Makes 2 servings.

ROASTED PEPPER SANDWICHES
(150 calories per serving)

Roasting, rather than grilling, adds tons of satisfying crunch to your cheese sandwich while skipping the extra fat. These toasted sandwiches with cheese have a lot of spiciness in every bite.

Ingredients:

- 2 slices of low-calorie bell pepper

- V2 cup of fresh arugula leaf cheese

- 4 thin slices of fresh tomato

- 4 slices of low-calorie whole-grain bread

Instructions:

1. Preheat the oven to 350 degrees F.

2. Place 1 slice of cheese on each of the 2 slices of bread; Cover each with 2 slices of tomato and half of the arugula. Cover with the remaining bread slices and place the sandwiches on a baking tray in the center of the oven.

3. Roast 4 minutes, then flip and roast an additional 2 to 3 minutes, or until the bread is golden and the cheese has melted. Cut cad

CHAPTER FIVE

FAST MONTH DAY MEAL PLAN

Each short day includes two of the recipes from Chapter 4, plus some delicious snacks from the list below. Women will consume 500 calories per day, while men will consume 600 per day.

You are not limited to eating food for breakfast or dinner. You are free to change your meals. For example, during the first week, day n. 1, you will have Tomato Parmesan Egg Toast, Chicken Breast Curry Wrap, and finger foods totaling 100 calories (for women) or 200 calories (for men). If you want to have a snack for breakfast and meals for lunch and dinner, that's fine.

If you want to have the Egg Parmesan Toast for breakfast, the chicken wrap for dinner, and your snacks the next day, that's fine too. For this reason, diet plans are not broken down into specific times of the day but into meals and snacks. This makes it much easier to plan your fasting day meals to suit your schedule and keeps you from getting lost.

Each fasting day, you will have two meals and two snacks. Men simply need to double their snack portions to get the required number of calories per day. Feel free to choose the items from the list of extra 50-calorie foods and snacks below that appeal to you.

On all fasting days, permitted drinks are limited to water, unsweetened hot or iced tea, and black coffee.

WEEK 1 PLAN

Fasting day 1

- First meal (150 calories): Egg toast and tomato parmesan (# 2)

- Second meal (250 calories): Curried Chicken Breast Wrap (# 3)

- Snacks (50 calories each): ½ medium apple, baked and sprinkled with cinnamon; 1 slice of crusty bread with 1 ounce of cottage cheese

Fasting day 2

- First meal (200 calories): protein sweet potatoes (# 5)

- Second meal (200 calories): Chicken with sesame lemon and asparagus (# 10)

- Snacks (50 calories each): ½ frozen medium banana; 1 can of raisins

WEEK 2 PLAN

Fasting day 1

- First meal (200 calories): Grilled chicken salad with poppy seed dressing (# 12)

- Meal 2 (200 calories): Baked salmon fillets with

tomatoes and mushrooms (# 4)

- Snacks (50 calories each): 4 oz unsweetened applesauce sprinkled with cinnamon; 1½ cup air popcorn

Fasting day 2

First meal (250 calories): Hearty shrimp and kale soup (# 8)

- Meal 2 Meals (150 calories): Omelette with spinach and Swiss cheese (# 11)

- Snacks (50 calories each): ½ cup strawberries with two tablespoons of fat-free vanilla yogurt; ½ cup shelled edamame with sea salt

WEEK 3 PLAN

Fasting day 1

- First meal (250 calories): Quinoa with black bean and sweet potato curry (# 15)

- Meal 2 (150 calories): Quick Bok Choy Shrimp Miso Soup (# 13)

- Snacks (50 calories each): 1 medium peach; 2 tablespoons of hummus with 2 sliced red peppers

Fasting day 2

- First meal (200 calories): Roasted Halibut with garlic spinach (# 14)

- Meal 2 Meals (200 calories): Penne with vegetables (# 7)

- Snacks (50 calories each): 1 small stalk of celery with ½ tablespoon of almond butter; 2 slices of avocado in lime juice

WEEK 4 PLAN

Fasting day 1

- First meal (250 calories): Greek breakfast wrap (# 1)

- Meal 2 (150 calories): Avocado fennel salad with balsamic vinaigrette (# 6)

- Aperitifs (50 calories each): 10 frozen grapes; 1 light Babybel cheese

Fasting day 2

First meal (250 calories): pork loin chop with mango sauce

(Second meal (150 calories): grilled pepper sandwiches

Snacks (50 calories each): 12 cherries; ½ small apple with 1 teaspoon of almond butter

The 50 Calories Food Supplements and Snacks List

Your fasting meals will be supplemented with healthy foods from this list. Each of these items contains 50 calories or a little less. Men simply need to double their portions to meet their highest daily needs (600 total calories).

You can also use this list to complement any no-fast day meal plans you create with the healthy recipes in Chapters 8, 9, and 10. This simple way to count calories and control your portions makes it much easier to keep track of. plan for a long time. -finished.

- Apple: ½ medium, baked and sprinkled with cinnamon

- Apple: ½ small, with 1 teaspoon of almond butter

- Apple (Granny Smith): 1 small

- Applesauce (unsweetened): 4 ounces, sprinkled with cinnamon • Avocado: 2 slices, with lemon juice

- Babybel cheese (light): 1 turn

- Small carrots: ½ cup, with 1 tablespoon of ranch fat-free • Banana: ½ medium, frozen

- Blueberries ½ cup, with 2 teaspoons of plain fat-free yogurt

- Brown rice cake: 1 cake, with ½ teaspoon of almond butter

- Melon (chopped): ½ cup, with 2 tablespoons of fat-free cottage cheese

- Celery branch: 1 small, with ½ tablespoon of almond butter

- Cherries: 12 whole

- Cherry tomatoes: 16 whole

- Crispbread: 1 slice, with 1 oz of cottage cheese

- Dill pickles: 6 medium

- Edamame (peeled): ½ cup, with sea salt

- Grapes (frozen): 10 whole

- Greek yogurt (fat-free): ½ cup, with ½ cup blueberries

- Green olives (pitted): 10 whole

- Hummus: 2 tablespoons, with 2 sliced red peppers

- Miso soup (instant): 1 cup, with ¼ cup frozen spinach

- Fishing: 1 medium

- Popcorn (with air): 1½ cup

- Raisins: 1 mini-box

- Red grapefruit: ½ large

- Strawberries: ½ cup, with 2 tablespoons of fat-free vanilla yogurt

- Strawberries: 12 whole

- Mandarin: 1 whole

- Tomato: 1 large, with 1 tablespoon of Parmesan

- Turkey breast: 2 slices (1 ounce) wrapped in lettuce leaves • Vegetable juice

- mixture: 6 ounces

CHAPTER SIX

RECIPES FOR NON -FASTING DAYS

BREAKFAST

A Note on No-Fast Day Recipes: No-Fast Day Recipes are low in calories but suitable for guests or the whole family, so we've created most of them to make four servings. You can halve the ingredients or freeze extra portions for easy reheating on another day if you want.

PEACH AND NUT PARFAITS

These parfaits may look pretty, but they're even healthier than they look. Nuts add omega-3 fatty acids and fiber and are crunchy, and Greek yogurt has up to fourteen grams of protein per cup.

Ingredients:

- 4 medium peaches, sliced

- ½ cup unsalted walnuts, chopped

- 4 containers (6 ounces) of vanilla Greek yogurt

- Divide the ingredients among four dessert or parfait plates. Start with a layer of peaches; then add a tablespoon of yogurt then a pinch of nuts.

- Makes 4 servings.

EGG SANDWICHES WITH SALMON AND TOMATO

This breakfast sandwich is so much healthier and more filling than anything you can buy while driving; It is also much tastier, but its preparation only takes a few minutes.

Ingredients:

- 4 light multigrain English muffins

- 1 teaspoon of olive oil

- 6 ounces of canned pink salmon

- 1 cup diced tomatoes

- 8 large eggs, beaten

- ½ teaspoon of salt

- ¼ teaspoon freshly ground black pepper

- 1 cup of fresh arugula

Instructions:

1. Toast the English muffins while you prepare the eggs.

2. In a medium skillet, heat olive oil over medium-high heat. Add the Salmon and tomatoes to the pan and sauté, frequently stirring, for 4 minutes.

3. Pour the eggs on top, season with salt and pepper, and stir, frequently stirring, for about 2 minutes, or until the eggs are set.

4. Arrange the English muffin halves on 4 plates and top

each bottom half with a quarter of the egg mixture. Top with arugula and the other half of the muffin.

5. Makes 4 servings.

COCOA BANANA BREAKFAST SHAKE

This shake only takes seconds to prepare, but it's packed with nutrients. Greek yogurt provides a healthy dose of protein, and bananas are a great source of potassium.

Ingredients:

- 24 ounces of vanilla Greek yogurt

- 2 medium bananas, cut into pieces

- 1 teaspoon of honey

- 2 tablespoons of unsweetened cocoa powder

- ½ cup of skimmed milk

- ½ cup of ice cubes

Instructions:

- Put the yogurt and bananas in a blender and blend over high heat until the bananas are smooth. Add honey, cocoa, and milk, and mix again until well incorporated.

- Add ice and mix again, pulsing as needed, until smooth and thick.

- Makes 4 servings.

WHOLE WHEAT BLUEBERRY NUT PANCAKES

These pancakes are a delicious way to start the day. Blueberries are tangy but sweet, and nuts add crunch and texture to this comforting classic.

Ingredients:

- ½ cup of fresh blueberries

- ½ teaspoon of pure vanilla extract

- ¾ cup whole wheat flour

- 1¼ cup low-fat milk

- 2 tablespoons of sugar

- 1 large egg, beaten

- 1 tablespoon of baking powder

- ½ cup of chopped walnuts

- ¼ teaspoon of salt

- 1 tablespoon of coconut oil, divided

- ½ teaspoon ground nutmeg

Instructions:

1. In a small bowl, toss the blueberries with a handful of whole wheat flour, tossing well to coat.

2. In a large bowl, combine the remaining flour, sugar, baking powder, salt, and nutmeg, stirring to combine

well.

3. Add the vanilla, milk, and egg and stir to combine, but do not over mix. The dough should be a bit lumpy. Gently fold in the nuts and blueberries (with the flour) and set aside the dough for 10 minutes.

4. In a large, heavy-bottomed pan, heat about ½ teaspoon of coconut oil over medium heat. Pour enough batter into the pan to make a 6-inch pancake. Cook for about 2 minutes or until the edges are bubbling, then flip the pancake and cook 1 minute more. Transfer to a plate and cover to keep warm while you prepare the rest of the pancakes. Add additional coconut oil to the pan as needed.

5. To serve, place 2 pancakes on each plate and garnish with hot maple syrup, honey, or molasses.

6. Makes 4 servings.

SCRAMBLED EGG TACOS

Finding fast food alternatives for breakfast can be difficult, but this recipe is a great one to try. It's full of southwestern flavor but low in fat and calories.

Ingredients:

- 8 whole wheat tortillas (6 inches)

- 12 large eggs, beaten

- 1 teaspoon of olive oil

- 1 cup thick sweet sauce

- 2 green onions, chopped

- 1 cup low-fat shredded cheddar cheese

- ½ teaspoon of Cayenne cheese

Instructions:

1. Place the tortillas on a plate, cover with a damp paper towel, and microwave for 30 to 45 seconds, or until warm and supple. Cover with a second plate or pot lid to keep warm.

2. In a large, heavy-bottomed skillet, heat olive oil over medium heat. Add the chives and sauté for 1 minute. Add the cayenne pepper to the eggs and pour them into the pan. Stir, stirring continuously, until eggs are set, about 5 minutes.

3. Divide the egg mixture evenly among the tortillas, top the tortillas with two tablespoons of salsa and cheddar cheese, and fold the tacos in half.

4. Makes 4 servings (2 tacos each).

HERBAL AND SWISS FRITTATA

This frittata looks like something you would see in a restaurant, but it only takes a few minutes to prepare. You'll love the layered flavors, thanks to the mild Swiss cheese and fresh herbs.

Ingredients:

- 2 teaspoons of olive oil

- 8 large eggs, beaten

- ½ teaspoon of salt

- ½ teaspoon of freshly ground black pepper

- 2 teaspoons of chopped fresh parsley

- 2 teaspoons of chopped fresh marjoram

- 1 teaspoon of fresh basil, minced

- ½ cup grated low-fat Swiss cheese

Instructions:

1. Preheat the oven to 375 degrees F.

2. Heat olive oil in a large skillet over high heat. Pour the eggs, distributing them evenly in the pan, season with salt and pepper.

3. Remove the pan from the heat and sprinkle the parsley, marjoram, and basil evenly on top of the eggs. Top with Swiss cheese.

4. Place pan in the oven center and bake 18 to 22 minutes or until a toothpick inserted in the center comes out clean.

5. To serve, cut into four wedges and serve hot.

6. Makes 4 servings.

VANILLA ALMOND PROTEIN SHAKE

This breakfast shake is packed with protein and healthy fats to keep you going on even the most challenging mornings. It's a great way to make breakfast on the go - just pour it into a travel mug and drink it on the go.

Ingredients:

- 2 cups of cold water

- 4 scoops of unflavored whey protein powder

- ¼ cup almond butter

- 2 tablespoons of honey

- ½ teaspoon of almond extract

- ½ teaspoon ground nutmeg

- 10 ice cubes

Instructions:

1. In a blender, combine cold water, protein powder, almond butter, honey, almond extract, and nutmeg. Blend over high heat for about 30 seconds or until smooth.

2. Add ice cubes and mix again until thick and creamy. Drink immediately.

3. Makes 2 servings.

SCRAMBLED EGGS WITH MUSHROOMS AND ONIONS

This egg dish cooks quickly but has a flavor that will ask you to slow down and taste. It also makes a hearty sandwich filling. If you have to eat your breakfast on the go, a whole wheat pita is a right choice.

Ingredients:

- 1 teaspoon of olive oil

- 1 cup sliced fresh mushrooms

- ¼ cup finely sliced yellow onion

- 1 tablespoon chopped fresh tarragon

- ½ cup chopped fresh parsley

- ½ teaspoon of salt

- ½ teaspoon of freshly ground black pepper

- 8 large eggs, beaten

Instructions:

1. In a large, heavy-bottomed skillet, heat olive oil over medium heat. Add the mushrooms, onion, tarragon, parsley, salt and pepper, and brown for 4 minutes, stirring occasionally.

2. Add eggs and stir, continually stirring, until cooked through, about 2 minutes. To serve, divide among 4 plates.

3. Makes 4 servings.

GRILLED FRUIT SALAD

Fruits don't always have to be raw; indeed, toasting or roasting fresh fruit brings out its natural sugars and intensifies its flavor. Double the recipe and use the leftovers as a garnish for chicken or seafood.

Ingredients:

- 8 slices of fresh or canned pineapple (unsweetened)

- 4 fresh peaches or nectarines, pitted and cut into 8 pieces each

- 8 slices (½ inch thick) of fresh honeydew melon

- 1 teaspoon of honey, heated for 30 seconds in the microwave

- ½ teaspoon of salt

Instructions:

1. Preheat the grill and line a baking sheet with foil.

2. Distribute the fruit in a single layer on the baking sheet and coat it with honey on both sides. Sprinkle salt on top and place the pan 3 inches below

3. The grill.

4. Grill for 3 minutes, turn each piece of fruit, then grill for 2 more minutes, or until the fruit is lightly browned around the edges.

5. Place 2 pineapple slices, 8 peach slices, and 2 melon slices on each of the 4 plates and serve hot.

6. Makes 4 servings.

HEARTY HOT CEREALS WITH RED FRUITS

Whole grains aren't just right for the heart; they are also ideal for your height. The high fiber content keeps them filled and provides slow, steady energy for your day. The addition of berries and nuts in this recipe makes it incredibly filling.

Ingredients:

- 4 cups of water

- 2 tablespoons of honey

- ½ teaspoon of salt

- ½ cup of fresh blueberries

- 2 cups of whole oats

- ½ cup of fresh raspberries

- ½ cup of chopped nuts

- 1 cup of skimmed milk

- 2 teaspoons of flax seeds

Instructions:

1. In a medium saucepan, bring water to a boil over high heat and add salt.

2. Add the oats, nuts, and flax seeds, then reduce the heat to low and cover. Bake for 16 to 20 minutes or until oatmeal reaches desired consistency.

3. Divide the oatmeal among 4 deep bowls and top each with 2 tablespoons of blueberries and raspberries. Add ¼ cup of milk to each bowl and serve.

4. Makes 4 servings.

EASY GRANOLA BARS

This recipe is so much better for you than any commercial granola bar, often loaded with high fructose corn syrup and less healthy grains. These bars cook in a jiffy and keep in an airtight container for up to a week, that is, if they last that long.

Ingredients:

- 1 teaspoon of coconut oil

- ¼ cup of melted coconut oil

- 1 cup of walnut pieces

- ½ cup of almond butter

- 1 cup of raw pumpkin seeds

- ½ cup of raw honey

- 1 cup of chopped walnuts

- ¼ teaspoon of pure vanilla extract

- 1 cup of dried cranberries

- ½ teaspoon of salt

- 1 cup of dried apricots, chopped

- 1 teaspoon of ground cinnamon

- 1 cup unsweetened coconut flakes

Instructions:

1. Preheat the oven to 325 degrees F. Grease a 9 by a 13-inch baking dish with 1 teaspoon of coconut oil and set aside.

2. In a large bowl, combine nuts, pumpkin seeds, pecans, blueberries, apricots, coconut flakes and mix well.

3. In a small saucepan over low heat, combine the melted coconut oil, almond butter, honey, vanilla, salt, cinnamon, and heat until the honey dissolves.

4. Transfer the nut mixture to the baking sheet, pressing down to spread evenly.

5. Pour the honey mixture evenly over the top.

6. Bake for 35 to 40 minutes or until golden brown. Allow the mixture to cool to room temperature before cutting it into equal bars. Store in an airtight container for up to 1 week.

7. Makes 1 dozen bars.

BANANA NUT POPSICLES

A healthy breakfast doesn't have to be hot; in fact, it is frozen. Prepare a bunch of these popsicles ahead of time and keep them in the freezer. They also make a great after-school gift. Children love them!

Ingredients:

- 4 large, freshly ripe bananas

- 2 tablespoons of raw honey

- 4 ice cream sticks

- ¾ cup of chopped nuts

- ½ cup of almond butter

Instructions:

1. Peel and cut one end of each banana and insert a popsicle stick into the cut end.

2. In a small bowl, whisk together almond butter and honey, microwave for 10 to 15 seconds, or until slightly diluted. Pour onto a sheet of waxed paper or aluminum foil and spread with a spatula.

3. On another piece of waxed paper or aluminum foil, layout the chopped nuts: line a small baking sheet or large plate with the third piece of waxed paper or aluminum foil.

4. Roll each banana first in the honey mixture until well coated, then in the nuts until completely covered, pressing gently down so that the nuts adhere.

5. Place each finished banana on the baking sheet. When all the bananas are covered, but the leaf in the freezer for at least 2 hours. For long-term storage, transfer the frozen bananas to a resealable plastic bag.

Produces 4 pops.

- ¼ cup dried cranberries

- ¼ cup of your favorite homemade or store-bought balsamic vinaigrette

- ½ orange pepper, chopped

- ½ yellow pepper, chopped

LUNCH

A Note on No-Fast Day Recipes: No-Fast Day Recipes are low in calories but suitable for guests or the whole family, so we've created most of them to make four servings. You can halve the ingredients or freeze extra portions for easy reheating on another day if you want.

SHRIMP AND BLUEBERRY SALAD

Dried cranberries add a tangy touch of flavor to this fresh shrimp salad. Using steamed shrimp from your seafood counter makes this a quick meal to prepare.

Ingredients:

- 1 large dozen (26-30 units) cooked

- ½ cup sliced red onion shrimps, peeled and deveined

- ¼a cup of lemon juice

- ¼ teaspoon ground cumin

- ¼ teaspoon of paprika

- 2 cups chopped romaine lettuce

Instructions:

1. In a small bowl, combine the shrimp with lime juice, cumin, and paprika and stand for 30 minutes in the refrigerator. Drain.

2. In a large bowl, combine lettuce, onion, peppers, and blueberries until well combined.

3. Add the marinated shrimp and balsamic vinaigrette and stir again. Divide among 4 salad plates and serve.

4. Makes 4 servings.

POCKETS OF TUNA AND BEAN SALAD

This light but the hearty recipe is ideal for weekday lunches. It packs well, and the flavor gets better the longer you have the opportunity to sit down, so make the salad the night before and put it in a pita pocket, then in your lunch bag in the morning.

Ingredients:

- 4 bags of whole wheat pita

- 1 can (6 ounces) tuna packed in water, drained

- ½ (15 ounces) pinto beans, rinsed and drained

- ¼ cup white onion, minced

- 2 tablespoons of light mayonnaise

- 1 teaspoon of spicy brown mustard

- ½ teaspoon of celery seeds

- ½ teaspoon of freshly ground black pepper

- 1 cup chopped romaine lettuce

Instructions:

1. If the pitas are not sliced, cut them so that there is a pocket-like opening, being careful not to cut the sides or the bottom.

2. In a small bowl, combine the tuna, pinto beans, onion, mayonnaise, mustard, celery seeds, and pepper; mix well.

3. Divide the lettuce among the pita pockets, then top each with a quarter of the tuna salad.

4. Makes 4 servings.

CHICKEN BREAST WITH ROASTED SUMMER VEG

This recipe heats up nicely, making it on the weekends or overnight and wrap in individual containers to take out for lunch during the week. Experiment with other seasonal vegetables to vary the flavors.

Ingredients:

- 4 skinless chicken breasts (4 to 5 ounces)

- 1 teaspoon and 1 tablespoon of olive oil, divided

- 1 teaspoon of salt, divided

- ½ teaspoon freshly ground black pepper, divided

- ½ teaspoon of ground turmeric

- 1 medium zucchini, thinly sliced

- 2 yellow squash, thinly sliced

- 1 medium white onion, sliced ½ inch thick

- 1 pint of cherry tomatoes

- 1 teaspoon of dried parsley

- 1 teaspoon of dried oregano

Instructions:

1. Preheat the oven to 400 degrees F and line a baking sheet with foil.

2. Rub both sides of the chicken breasts with 1 teaspoon of olive oil and season with ½ teaspoon of salt, ¼ teaspoon of pepper, and turmeric. Place the chicken in the pan.

3. In a medium bowl, combine zucchini, squash, onion, and tomatoes. Add the parsley and oregano, then drizzle with the remaining tablespoon of olive oil. Mix the vegetables well until evenly coated and distribute around the chicken breasts in the pan.

4. Bake in the oven center for 15 minutes, turn the chicken, toss the vegetables, then bake for an additional 10 to 12 minutes, or until the chicken juices run clear.

5. To serve, place 1 breast on each plate and garnish with 1/4 of the vegetables.

6. Makes 4 servings.

EASY CHICKEN PASTA SOUP

Boil the pasta a day or two before and after draining it, place it in a resealable bag in the refrigerator until ready to use. This little prep work makes this soup a lunch that only takes ten minutes.

Ingredients:

- 3 cups of chicken broth

- 1 teaspoon of fresh thyme leaves

- 1 cup of frozen green beans

- ½ teaspoon of salt

- 1 cup of frozen sliced carrots

- ¼ teaspoon of freshly ground black

- 1 can (6 ounces) grated chicken, drained with pepper

- 1 cup of mini pasta with cooked shells

- 1 teaspoon of chopped fresh tarragon

- ½ cup grated Parmesan

Instructions:

1. In a large pot, bring the chicken broth to a boil over high heat. Add the green beans and carrots and reduce the heat to medium. Cover and simmer for 5 minutes.

2. Add the chicken, tarragon, and thyme, salt, pepper,

and simmer for another 4 minutes. Remove the pan from the heat and add the cooked pasta.

3. To serve, divide among 4 bowls and garnish with Parmesan.

4. Makes 4 servings.

AVOCADOS STUFFED WITH SEAFOOD.

It's a great light lunch, especially in the warmer months. You can make the filling up to three days in advance and simply assemble the dish when you're ready to eat.

Ingredients:

- 2 medium tomatoes, diced

- 1 tablespoon of light Italian vinaigrette

- 2 cups chopped iceberg lettuce

- 1 tablespoon of mayonnaise

- 4 slices of turkey bacon

- ½ cup of plain croutons

- 2 avocados

- 1 teaspoon of lemon juice

Instructions:

1. In a medium bowl, combine shrimp, crabmeat, celery, bell pepper, onion, and chives; mix well.

2. In a small bowl, combine mayonnaise, yogurt, dry

mustard, parsley, and black pepper, and stir with a fork until combined.

3. Mix mayonnaise mixture with seafood filling until blended.

4. Cut the avocados in half, remove the bones and clean the pulp with the lemon juice. Fill each avocado half with a quarter of the seafood filling and serve.

5. Makes 4 servings.

CHOPPED BLT SALAD

This salad lets you savor all the BLT sandwich's classic flavors without going overboard on the fat and calories. Using turkey bacon and croutons (instead of bread) goes a long way in making this a healthier way to have a BLT.

Ingredients:

- 2 chives, sliced

- ½ teaspoon of freshly ground black pepper

- ½ red pepper, chopped

- ½ red onion, chopped

- 2 tablespoons of chopped fresh parsley

- ¼ teaspoon of dry mustard

- 8 ounces of grated imitation crab meat,

- 1 tablespoon of chopped plain yogurt

- 1 stalk of celery, finely chopped

- 1 cup cooked cocktail shrimp

- 2 tablespoons of light mayonnaise

Instructions:

1. Heat turkey bacon in the microwave according to package directions.

2. Let drain on absorbent paper and let cool for 5 minutes.

3. Meanwhile, combine lettuce, tomatoes, and croutons in a large bowl.

4. In a small cup, mix the mayonnaise and the Italian dressing (it will be thick).

5. Crumble the bacon and add it to the salad. Pour the dressing over everything and toss well until the salad is coated. Divide among 2 plates and serve.

6. Makes 2 servings.

ENERGIZING GREEN SMOOTHIE

Even if you don't have time for lunch, you will still have time to consume plenty of vitamins and minerals in the form of this smoothie. The healthy fat in the avocado and the fiber in vegetables means you'll feel fuller too.

Ingredients:

- 1 medium cucumber, peeled and chopped

- 2 cups of fresh baby spinach

- ½ cup of fresh parsley

- 1 cup of carrot juice

- ½ teaspoon of salt

- 2 pinches of hot red pepper sauce

- ½ avocado, chopped

Instructions:

1. Combine cucumber, spinach, parsley, carrot juice, salt, and hot sauce in a blender and mix over high heat until smooth.

2. Add avocado and mix on medium speed until smooth. Divide among 4 glasses and serve immediately.

3. Makes 4 servings.

GRILLED HAM, SWISS, AND ARUGULA SANDWICHES

This grilled sandwich leaves out the fat of typical grilled ham and cheese and adds a lot more crunch. Served with a light soup or salad, it's a delicious and healthy lunch meal.

Ingredients:

- 8 slices of low-calorie whole wheat bread

- 2 teaspoons Dijon mustard

- 1 pound (approximately 16 slices) lean deli ham, thinly sliced

- 8 slices low-fat Swiss cheese

- 1 cup of fresh arugula

Instructions:

1. Preheat the oven to 350 degrees F.

2. Spread Dijon mustard on four slices of bread and garnish with about 4 slices of ham and 2 slices of cheese.

3. Top each with ¼ cup arugula and place remaining bread slices on sandwiches. Bake in the oven center for 5 minutes, turn it over, then bake for another 3 minutes, or until the bread is golden brown and the cheese is melted. Cut each sandwich in half and serve hot.

4. Makes 4 servings.

QUICK AND LIGHT WHITE BEAN CHILI

This chili doesn't take long (and just one pan) to cook and tastes even better the next day. It also freezes well, making a double batch to portion and keep in the freezer on busy days.

- 1 teaspoon of olive oil

- 1 pound of freshly ground turkey breast

- 1 teaspoon of chili powder

- 1 teaspoon of salt

- ½ teaspoon of freshly ground black pepper

- ½ teaspoon of ground cumin

- 1 cup chopped white onion

- 2 tablespoons of chopped fresh coriander

- 2 cans (15 ounces) large Nordic beans, undrained

- 2 cups chicken broth

Instructions:

1. In a medium-heavy saucepan, heat olive oil over medium-high heat. Add the turkey, chili powder, salt, pepper, and cumin and sauté and sauté for 7 to 8 minutes, often chopping with a spatula, until the turkey is cooked through.

2. Add onion and sauté 1 more minute before adding cilantro, beans with liquid, and chicken broth. Bring to a boil, then reduce the heat to low, cover, and simmer for 15 minutes. Divide among 4 soup bowls and serve hot.

3. Makes 4 servings.

VEGETABLE MARKET REVOLT

There is nothing wrong with breakfast for lunch. This dish cooks in minutes and will keep you going all day.

Ingredients:

- 1 teaspoon of olive oil

- ½ red pepper, diced

- ½ cup chopped white onion

- 1 cup sliced fresh mushrooms

- ½ teaspoon of salt

- ¼ teaspoon freshly ground black pepper

- 8 large eggs, beaten

Instructions:

1. In a large, heavy-bottomed skillet, heat olive oil over medium heat. Add the bell pepper, onion, mushrooms, salt, and pepper and sauté for 5 minutes, stirring frequently.

2. Pour the eggs on top and stir, stirring continuously, for about 3 minutes, or until the eggs are set. Divide among 4 plates and serve hot.

3. Makes 4 servings.

EGGPLANT, HUMMUS, AND GOAT CHEESE SANDWICHES

Grilled eggplant slices replace cold cuts, and hummus adds protein and fiber while replacing mayonnaise. Try this classic Greek recipe and bring a Mediterranean touch to your lunch table.

Ingredients:

- 1 medium eggplant, cut into ½ inch thick slices

- Sea salt

- 2 tablespoons of olive oil

- Freshly ground black pepper

- 5 to 6 tablespoons of hummus

- 4 slices of whole-wheat toast

- 1 cup of young spinach leaves

- 2 ounces of goat cheese or feta cheese, softened

Instructions:

1. Preheat a gas or charcoal grill over medium-high heat.

2. Season both sides of the sliced eggplant with salt and stand for 20 minutes to extract the bitter juice. Rinse the eggplant and pat it dry with a paper towel.

3. Brush the eggplant with olive oil and season to taste with S&P.

4. Grill eggplants until lightly charred on both sides but still slightly firm in the middle, 3 to 4 minutes per side.

5. Spread the hummus on 2 slices of bread and garnish with spinach leaves, goat cheese, and eggplant. Garnish with the remaining pieces of bread and serve.

6. To reheat.

7. Makes 2 servings.

DINNER

A Note on No-Fast Day Recipes: No-Fast Day Recipes are low in calories but suitable for guests or the whole family, so we've created most of them to make four servings. You can halve the ingredients or freeze extra portions for easy reheating on another day if you want.

SPICY ORANGE CHICKEN BREAST

This recipe offers both speed and flavor. It's a great dish to make on busy evenings. Served with a green salad and quinoa or brown rice, it's a light yet satisfying meal.

Ingredients:

- 1 teaspoon of olive oil

- 4 skinless chicken breasts (4 to 5 ounces)

- 1 teaspoon of paprika

- ½ teaspoon of salt

- ¼ teaspoon freshly ground black pepper

- 1 teaspoon of chopped fresh thyme

- 1 teaspoon of chopped fresh rosemary

- 1 tablespoon of unsweetened concentrated orange juice

- 2 tablespoons of chopped fresh parsley

Instructions:

1. Preheat the oven to 400 degrees F and line a baking dish with foil.

2. Distribute the olive oil to the bottom of the plate.

3. Arrange the chicken breasts on the plate, turn them to coat them with oil, and season with paprika, salt, pepper, thyme, and rosemary.

4. Bake for 15 minutes, then turn the chicken and brush with the orange juice concentrate. Bake for an additional 15 to 20 minutes or until the chicken juices run clear.

5. Garnish with parsley before serving.

6. Makes 4 servings.

GRILLED SHRIMP AND BLACK BEAN SALAD

This recipe is excellent to use when you have company for dinner. No one will think it is low in calories!

Ingredients:

- 1 teaspoon of lime zest (about ½ lime)

- ¼ cup of freshly squeezed lemon juice

- 3 tablespoons of olive oil

- 2 tablespoons chopped fresh basil

- 2 tablespoons minced fresh oregano

- 1 teaspoon of freshly ground black pepper

- ½ teaspoon of salt

- 2 cans (15 ounces) black beans, rinsed and drained

- 1 cup diced tomatoes

- 1 cup diced green pepper

- ½ cup of green onions, chopped

- 24 large raw shrimps (21-25 units), peeled and deveined

1. In a medium bowl, combine lime zest and juice, olive oil, basil, oregano, pepper, and mix well. Measure 2 tablespoons in a small bowl and set aside.

2. Add salt, black beans, tomatoes, peppers, and onion to the medium bowl and mix well. Put in the refrigerator until ready to serve.

3. Preheat a flat grill to medium-high heat. Once hot, place the shrimp on the grill and drizzle with the reserved lemon juice mixture. Cook 3 minutes on one side, then turn over, bathe again and cook for another 3 minutes.

4. To serve, place 1/4 of the bean salad on each plate and top with 6 hot shrimp.

5. Makes 4 servings.

MAPLE GLAZED SALMON WITH MUSTARD

This is an incredibly delicious salmon recipe, especially considering how quick and easy it is to prepare. Add a baked sweet potato or brown rice, and you have a rich and tasty meal.

Ingredients:

- 4 salmon fillets (6 ounces) with skin ¾ inch thick

- 1 teaspoon of olive oil

- ½ teaspoon of salt

- ½ teaspoon of freshly ground black pepper

- 2 tablespoons of pure maple syrup

- ½ teaspoon of dry mustard

- 8 sprigs of fresh thyme

Instructions:
- Preheat a flat grill to medium-high heat.

- Brush salmon fillets on both sides with olive oil, season with salt and pepper, and place on the grill skin side down. Cook for 7 minutes.

- Meanwhile, mix the maple syrup and dry mustard with a fork.

- Flip the salmon fillets, spread with the maple mustard glaze, and garnish each with 2 sprigs of thyme. Grill 5 to 7 minutes longer or until fish flakes easily.

- To serve, use a spatula to transfer the fillets to 4 plates, leaving the thyme intact.

- Makes 4 servings.

TUSCAN BAKED BAR

The sea bass is a tasty, delicate, and flaky fish. This Tuscan-inspired recipe complements this sweet fish with fresh tomatoes, nuts, basil, and garlic flavors.

Ingredients:

- 4 sea bass fillets (6 oz) with skin

- 1 teaspoon of olive oil

- 1 cup finely chopped walnuts (use a food processor or blender)

- 2 teaspoons minced garlic

- 8 slices of yellow or orange tomatoes, ¼ inch thick

- 8 slices of ¼ inch thick red onion

- ½ cup fresh basil, chopped

- ½ teaspoon of salt

- ¼ teaspoon freshly ground black pepper

Instructions:

1. Preheat the oven to 400 degrees F and line a baking sheet with foil.

2. Brush both sides of the sea bass fillets with olive oil and dip them in the chopped nuts, completely covering the fillets. Place the steaks skin side down on the baking sheet. Spread the garlic over the fillets, then garnish the fish by alternating slices of tomato and onion. Sprinkle with basil and season with salt and pepper.

3. Bake for 12 to 14 minutes or until the fish flakes easily. To serve, use a spatula to transfer the fillets to 4 plates.

4. Makes 4 servings.

PORTOBELLO BURGERS

You don't have to be a vegetarian to enjoy these burgers made with luscious portobello mushrooms. They're deliciously different but just as satisfying as a traditional burger, without all the fat and calories. Cannellini beans hidden under the lids make them hearty enough even for the most hungry of diners.

Ingredients:

- 4 large Portobello mushroom caps (4 inches wide)

- 1½ teaspoon olive oil, divided

- ½ teaspoon of salt

- ¼ teaspoon freshly ground black pepper

- ½ teaspoon minced garlic

- ½ teaspoon of paprika

- 1 cup canned cannellini beans

- 4 slices (1 oz) low-fat mozzarella cheese

- 4 whole-wheat hamburger buns

- 4 large leaves of romaine lettuce

- 4 slices of fresh tomato

- 8 slices of red onion

Instructions:

1. Preheat the oven to 325 degrees F.

2. Rub the sides of the mushrooms with ½ teaspoon of olive oil and season with salt and pepper.

3. In a large skillet, heat the remaining 1 teaspoon of olive oil over medium-high heat. Add the mushrooms, cover, and sauté for 4 minutes.

4. Meanwhile, combine the garlic, paprika, and beans and cook in the microwave for 1 minute or lukewarm. Leave besides.

5. Flip the mushrooms and place 1 slice of mozzarella on each. Reduce the heat to a minimum.

6. Toast the hamburger buns in the oven for 5 minutes or until crispy.

7. Transfer to 4 plates. Top buns below with lettuce, tomato, and onion.

8. Pour a quarter of the bean mixture into a mound in the center of each bun and top with a mushroom cover. Add the rolls and serve.

9. Makes 4 servings.

SPINACH AND FLANK STEAK SALAD

Skirt steak is a lean, flavorful cut of meat that's ideal for a calorie-restricted diet. This recipe calls for the steak to be cooked over medium heat. The heart tends to be quite picky if you cook a lot more than that.

Ingredients:

- 1 pound of skirt steak, with no visible fat or tendons

- ¼ cup balsamic dressing (see Avocado and Fennel Salad with Balsamic Vinaigrette recipe for instructions), divided

- ½ teaspoon salt

- ½ teaspoon of freshly ground black pepper

- 3 cups chopped romaine lettuce

- 1 cup of young spinach leaves

- 1 pint of cherry tomatoes, cut in half

- ½ cup sweet yellow onion, thinly sliced

Instructions:

1. Preheat a flat grill over high heat until it boils.

2. Brush the flank steak with two tablespoons of balsamic vinaigrette, season with salt and pepper, and place on the grill. Cook 5 minutes, then turn and cook 10 more minutes, or until the steak is medium-rare.

3. Meanwhile, mix lettuce, spinach, tomatoes, and onion until blended. Then add the remaining 2 tablespoons

of the dressing. Mix well to coat and divide the salad among 4 plates.

4. Transfer the steak to a plate and let stand 10 minutes before thinly slicing on the diagonal.

5. Place a quarter of the sliced steak on each salad and serve.

6. Makes 4 servings.

GROUND CHICKEN

This variation of a traditional Latin dish uses leaner chicken instead of beef. It doesn't take away from the spiciness but reduces the fat and calories typically found in the traditional version. Make an extra batch to freeze for later.

Ingredients:

- 2 teaspoons of olive oil
- ½ cup chopped yellow onion
- 2 minced garlic cloves
- ½ pound of ground chicken
- ½ teaspoon of ground cumin
- ½ teaspoon of salt
- ¼ teaspoon freshly ground black pepper
- 2 tablespoons of red wine

- 1 cup chopped tomato

- 1 fresh jalapeño pepper, seeded and diced

- ¼ cup green olives with peppers, chopped

- 1 teaspoon of Worcestershire sauce

- ¼ cup fresh cilantro, chopped

- 1 teaspoon of fresh lime juice (about ½ lime)

Instructions:

1. In a large, heavy-bottomed pan, heat olive oil over medium-high heat. Add onion and garlic and sauté for 2 minutes, stirring frequently.

2. Add the chicken, cumin, salt, and pepper and cook for 5 to 6 minutes, frequently stirring to shred the chicken.

3. Add the wine to the pan to deglaze, scraping up the golden bits from the bottom. Add tomato, jalapeño, olives, and Worcestershire sauce; Reduce the heat to medium and simmer 6 to 8 minutes or until the mixture thickens.

4. To serve, pour into 4 bowls and finish with a squeeze of lemon and a pinch of cilantro.

5. Makes 4 servings.

FLORENTINE CHICKEN

In this riff of appropriate Florentine dishes, the chicken

breasts are treated with a delicious creamy sauce sprinkled with fresh spinach. Serve it to your guests; they won't know you're on a diet.

Ingredients:

- 1 teaspoon of olive oil

- 4 boneless, skinless chicken breasts

- ½ teaspoon of salt

- ¼ teaspoon freshly ground black pepper

- ¼ cup of dry white wine

- ¼ cup chopped yellow onion

- 1 cup sliced fresh mushrooms

- 1 cup frozen chopped spinach, thawed and drained

- ½ cup of chicken broth

- ¼ cup low-fat milk

- ¼ cup grated Parmesan

Instructions:

1. In a large, heavy-bottomed pan, heat olive oil over medium-high heat.

2. Season the chicken breasts on both sides with salt and pepper and sauté for 5 minutes. Flip the chicken and cook an additional 5 to 7 minutes, or until the juices run clear. Transfer to a plate and cover to keep warm.

3. Add the wine to the pan to deglaze it and scrape the golden pieces from the bottom.

4. Add the onion, mushrooms, spinach, and chicken broth and simmer for 10 to 15 minutes or until the sauce is reduced by half.

5. Reduce the heat to medium, add the milk, and heat until heated through, about 1 minute.

6. To serve, place 1 chicken breast on each plate, top with 1/4 of the sauce, and sprinkle with Parmesan.

7. Makes 4 servings.

EASY BLACK BEAN SOUP

Served with a fresh salad and a crunchy bun, this dish is a hearty comfort meal. You'll get all the flavors of traditional black bean soup but in much less time.

Ingredients:

- 2 (15 oz) cans of black beans

- ½ teaspoon chili powder

- 2 cups of chicken broth

- 1 cup finely sliced carrots

- ½ cup chopped yellow onion

- ½ teaspoon of garlic powder

- ½ teaspoon of ground cumin

- ½ teaspoon of salt

- ¼ teaspoon freshly ground black pepper

- 1 cup of plain yogurt

- ¼ cup sliced green onions

Instructions:

1. In a large saucepan over medium-high heat, combine the black beans, chicken broth, carrots, onion, garlic powder, cumin, chili powder, and salt. Mix well.

2. Bring the soup to a boil, reduce the heat to medium, cover and simmer for 20 minutes, stirring occasionally.

3. To serve, serve in 4 bowls, top with a dollop of yogurt and garnish with green onions.

4. Makes 4 servings.

HEARTY VEGETABLE SOUP

This soup is easy to prepare and contains only a wide variety of vegetables. It's a great soup to serve with a salad or sandwich on nights when you don't feel like cooking, so double and freeze the excess.

Ingredients:

- 1 teaspoon of olive oil

- 1 cup diced Yukon Gold potatoes

- ½ cup thinly sliced carrots

- ½ cup fresh green beans, cut into 1-inch pieces

- ½ cup chopped yellow onion

- 1 cup of fresh spinach leaves

- 3 cups of chicken broth

- ¼ cup chopped fresh parsley

- 1 tablespoon of chopped fresh rosemary

- ½ teaspoon of salt

- ¼ teaspoon freshly ground black pepper

Instructions:

1. In a large, heavy-bottomed pan, heat olive oil over medium-high heat. Add the potatoes, carrots, green beans, and onion and sauté for 5 minutes, stirring frequently. Remove from the heat.

2. Transfer the vegetables to a large saucepan over medium-high heat. Add the spinach, chicken broth, parsley, rosemary, salt, and pepper, and bring the soup to a boil. Reduce the heat to medium, cover, and simmer for 30 minutes.

3. To serve, serve in 4 bowls.

4. Makes 4 servings.

STUFFED ZUCCHINI WITH MUSHROOMS

Fresh zucchini and mushrooms seasoned with garlic, olive oil, parsley, and Italian herbs and spices hardly appear to be diet foods. These mushroom-stuffed zucchini tins are a simple and impressive dish that's low in calories but still filling. Serve with a piece of fish for dinner or serve just for lunch.

Ingredients:

- 2 tablespoons of olive oil

- 2 cups finely chopped mushrooms

- 2 garlic cloves, finely chopped

- 2 tablespoons of chicken broth

- 1 tablespoon finely chopped flat-leaf parsley

- 1 tablespoon Italian seasoning

- Sea salt

- Freshly ground black pepper

- 2 medium zucchini, halved lengthwise

- 1 tablespoon of water

Instructions:

1. Preheat the oven to 350 degrees F.

2. Heat a large skillet over medium heat and add olive oil. Add the mushrooms and cook until tender, about 4 minutes. Add the garlic and cook for another 2 minutes. Add the chicken broth and cook for another 3 to 4 minutes.

3. Add the parsley and Italian seasoning, then season with salt and pepper to taste. Stir well and remove from heat.

4. Remove the seeds and a little zucchini pulp and fill the halves with the mushroom mixture.

5. Place the zucchini in a saucepan and pour 1 tablespoon of water over the bottom.

6. Cover with foil and bake for 30 to 40 minutes, or until zucchini is tender. Transfer to 2 plates and serve immediately.

7. Makes 2 servings.

SPICY MEAT SKEWERS

Tender, juicy, and spicy, these skewers will make you happy to eat healthily. Further proof that eating lean doesn't have to taste bad!

Ingredients:

- ½ cup of lemon juice

- 1 teaspoon of salt

- 1 teaspoon of black pepper

- 1 clove of minced garlic

- ¼ teaspoon of red pepper flakes

- ¼ teaspoon of chopped rosemary

- ¼ teaspoon of chopped basil

- 1 pound of lean red meat, such as beef, venison, or bison, cut into bite-sized cubes

- 1 red onion, peeled, halved horizontally, and quartered vertically

- 1 pkg of cherry tomatoes

- 2 green peppers, cut into slices similar to onion

Instructions:

1. Mix the first seven ingredients.

2. Add the meat to a large zipped plastic bag and pour the lime and spice mixture over it. Let marinate for at least 20 minutes; the longer, the better.

3. Preheat the grill to medium / high heat when you are ready to make the kebabs. Thread the meat, onions, tomatoes, and peppers onto the skewers.

4. Grill, 1 to 3 minutes on each of four sides or until the steak reaches the desired temperature.

5. Makes 4 servings.

SNACKS

LIGHTLY ROASTED NUTS

These nuts are a great alternative to store-bought salty versions.

Ingredients:

- 200 g unsalted raw nuts, such as almonds or peanuts

- 1 tablespoon (15 ml) canola or olive oil 1 teaspoon

- (5 ml) paprika V2 teaspoon

- (2.5 ml) ground cumin V2 teaspoon

- (2.5 ml) ground cinnamon black pepper to taste

Instructions:

1. Preheat the oven to 180 ° C and line a baking tray with parchment paper or aluminium foil.

2. Place all ingredients in a bowl and stir well to cover the nuts with the oil and spices. Season with pepper.

3. Place them on the baking tray and bake for 10-15 minutes or until lightly browned. Stir the pan once or twice during the cooking time. Be careful not to burn them.

4. Let cool and serve about 1 cup (80 ml) per person as a snack or sprinkle over a salad for extra crunch.

RAISIN COOKIES

Homemade cookies are much better than store-bought cookies because you can control what they contain. These are lower in fat and sugar, making them a healthier alternative.

Ingredients:

- One cup (80 ml) of soft margarine in a tub 'One cup

- (80 ml) of sugar 2 eggs, beaten

- 1 teaspoon (5 ml) vanilla extract

- 1 teaspoon (5 ml) finely grated lemon zest

- 1 cup (250 ml) whole wheat flour

- 1 cup (250 ml) confectioner's flour 100 ml raisins

Instructions:

1. Preheat the oven to 180 ° C and line a baking tray with parchment paper.

2. Put margarine and sugar in a bowl and beat until light and fluffy.

3. Add the eggs one at a time, beating well after each addition.

4. Add the vanilla and lemon zest and stir in the flour and raisins. Stir until smooth. Roll into balls and place on the baking tray. Press down with a fork.

Bake for 15 minutes or until golden brown. Let cool on a rack and store in an airtight container. Serve 2-3 small biscuits as a snack.

PEANUT BUTTER STRIPS

Peanut butter is a delicious baking ingredient. This will help bind and flavor the mixture.

Ingredients:

- 2 cups (500 ml) oatmeal One cup

- (80 ml) honey 'One cup

- (80 ml) pitted dates, chopped 5 tablespoons

- (75 ml) peanut butter 1 egg, beaten

- One cup

- (60 ml) of sunflower oil 1 teaspoon

- (5 ml) ground cinnamon or spice mix

- 1 teaspoon (5 ml) vanilla extract

Instructions:

1. Preheat the oven to 180 ° C and lightly grease an 18 x 30 cm baking dish.

2. Put all ingredients in a bowl and mix until well blended.

3. Press mixture into a baking pan until evenly coated and bake for 10-15 minutes or until golden and crisp.

4. Cut into 20 warm slices. Let cool on a cooling rack and remove it from the can. Store in an airtight container for 3-4 days.

5. Serve 2 slices per person as a snack.

DATE AND CHOCOLATE BALLS

We all love chocolate, but we know that too much is not good for us. In this treatment, we combine dark chocolate with dates to make a healthier alternative.

Ingredients:

- V2 x 80 g dark chocolate cut into pieces

- 1 tablespoon (15 ml) of cocoa

- 3 tablespoons (45 ml) of low-fat milk

- 1 teaspoon (5 ml) vanilla extract

- 250 g unpitted dates, finely chopped

- 100 ml extra coconut and cocoa desiccated coconut to decorate with

Instructions:

1. Place the chocolate in a glass container and melt over boiling water. Make sure the container does not touch the water.

2. Mix the cocoa with a little milk into a paste and mix with the remaining milk and vanilla. Add a little of the melted chocolate to the milk mixture until smooth. Mix with the hot chocolate.

3. Add the dates and coconut. Spoon the mixture onto baking paper and sprinkle with coconut or cocoa, and set aside. You can also cool slightly and roll into balls. Roll the balls in coconut or extra cocoa, if you prefer. Let cool in the refrigerator. Serve 1-2 scoops as a treat.

BABY MARROW FRITS

Baby marrows are very versatile and add extra fibre and flavor to this snack.

Ingredients:

- 2 cups (375 ml) whole wheat flour 1 teaspoon (5 ml) baking powder

- 1 cup (250 ml) buttermilk or mesh

- 2 beaten eggs

- 4 courgettes, coarsely grated 6 tablespoons

- (90 ml), grated cheddar or mozzarella 2 tablespoons

- (30 ml) sunflower or olive oil for frying.

Instructions:

1. Add zucchini and cheese and mix to a thick batter.

2. Heat half the oil in a large frying pan and fry the tablespoons of the mixture until golden brown.

3. Flip and fry on the other side until golden and cooked through.

4. Drain on kitchen paper.

5. Repeat with the remaining mixture and more oil if needed. Serve 3 fritters per person as a snack.

APPLE AND BANANA MUFFINS

Baking is often associated with a lot of sugar and a lower nutritional value. No sugar is needed when making applesauce and using a ripe banana. The grated apple gives these delicious muffins flavor and texture.

Ingredients:

- Apple puree (for 250 ml)

- 4 apples, peeled and diced One cup

- (60 ml) water 2 teaspoons

- (10 ml) lemon juice Muffins

- One cup (125 ml) whole wheat flour One cup

- (125 ml) cake flour One tablespoon

- (7.5 ml) baking powder 1 teaspoon

- (5 ml) ground cinnamon 1 cup

- (250 ml) grated apple coarse One 125 ml prepared apple sauce

- 1 large ripe banana, mashed with a fork

- 2 beaten eggs

- 6 tablespoons (90 ml) sunflower or canola oil 1 teaspoon

- (5 ml) vanilla extract

Instructions:

1. Muffins: Preheat, the oven to 180 ° C., Place the muffin cups in the muffin tin, or grease the pan.

2. Mix all the dry ingredients and add the grated apple. Mix the remaining ingredients.

3. Mix the liquid ingredients with the dry ingredients

into a smooth dough. Be careful not to over mix it. Pour into muffin tins and bake for 25-30 minutes or until a skewer comes out clean.

4. Let cool on a cooling rack. Serve one muffin per person as a snack or in a lunch box.

FRESH FRUIT AND BUTTER DIP

This peanut butter dip even turns fruit snacks into low-fat quark with% cup (60ml) of natural fat tastiest! Peanut butter, add a slightly sweeter yogurt, and season with lemon juice and black pepper. Add yogurt flavor, making it ideal for snacks.

Ingredients:

- 3 tablespoons (45 ml) peanut butter

- 2 cups (125 ml) of low-fat yogurt

- 4 apples or pears, cut into wedges

- Put the peanut butter in a bowl and mix until slightly soft. Add the yogurt and mix well until smooth.

- Serve a peanut butter dip with fruit wedges as an afternoon snack. Peanut butter and fruit can control sweet cravings.

Popcorn

Homemade popcorn is a treat and the ideal filling for the lunch box. A healthier alternative to salty store-bought snacks like French fries, you can control the amount of salt and oil used at home.

- 1 teaspoon (5 ml) of sunflower oil

- V2 cup (125 ml) of popcorn seeds One teaspoon (1.2 ml) of salt

- 2 teaspoons (10 ml) of dried herbs, origanum, or paprika

Instructions:

1. Place the oil in a large saucepan with a lid and turn to coat the bottom of the pan with oil.

2. Sprinkle grains in an even layer on the bottom of the pot. Cover with a lid and heat over medium heat.

3. Do not leave the pan unattended when the popcorn kernels start to pop. Remove the pan from the heat if more than 2 seconds elapse between each 'pop.' Do not remove the cap until it will no longer open.

4. Mix together the salt and herbs or spices and sprinkle over the hot popcorn. Stir and serve immediately.

CONCLUSION

Intermittent fasting is a diet that involves regular, short-term fasting. The best types for women over 50 include daily fasting for 14 to 16 hours, the 5: 2 diet, or modified fasting every other day.

While intermittent fasting is beneficial for heart health, diabetes, and weight loss, some evidence may have adverse effects on reproduction and blood sugar levels in some women.

That said, modified versions of intermittent fasting seem safe for most women and perhaps a more suitable option than longer or stricter fasts. If you are a woman looking to lose weight or improve her health, intermittent fasting is something to consider.

- If you enjoyed *Intermittent fasting for Women over 50*, please do me a favor! Let me know your thoughts by leaving a short review, I'd really appreciate that. Thank you ☺ -

Lightning Source UK Ltd.
Milton Keynes UK
UKHW021921040321
379813UK00003B/323